Includes **meal plans, recipes,** and **nutritional information**

The **Daily**

Vegan
Planner

12 WEEKS
to a Complete Vegan Diet Transition

JOLINDA HACKETT
author of *The Everything® Vegan Cookbook*, with **Nicole Cormier, RD, LDN**

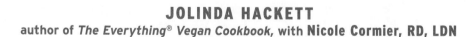

Adams media
AVON, MASSACHUSETTS

Published by
Adams Media, a division of F+W Media, Inc.
57 Littlefield Street, Avon, MA 02322. U.S.A.
www.adamsmedia.com

Contains material adapted and abridged from *The Everything*® *Vegan Cookbook* by
Jolinda Hackett with Lorena Novak Bull, RD, copyright © 2010 by F+W Media, Inc.,
ISBN 10: 1-4405-0216-1, ISBN 13: 978-1-4405-0216-3.

ISBN-10: 1-4405-2998-1
ISBN-13: 978-1-4405-2998-6
eISBN-10: 1-4405-3124-2
eISBN-13: 978-1-4405-3124-8

Printed in the United States of America.

10   9   8   7   6   5   4   3   2   1

Library of Congress Cataloging-in-Publication Data
is available from the publisher.

This publication is designed to provide accurate and authoritative information with
regard to the subject matter covered. It is sold with the understanding that the publisher
is not engaged in rendering legal, accounting, or other professional advice. If legal
advice or other expert assistance is required, the services of a competent professional
person should be sought.
—From a *Declaration of Principles* jointly adopted by a Committee of the American
Bar Association and a Committee of Publishers and Associations

Many of the designations used by manufacturers and sellers to distinguish their product
are claimed as trademarks. Where those designations appear in this book and Adams
Media was aware of a trademark claim, the designations have been printed with initial
capital letters.

This book is intended as general information only, and should not be used to diagnose
or treat any health condition. In light of the complex, individual, and specific nature
of health problems, this book is not intended to replace professional medical advice.
The ideas, procedures, and suggestions in this book are intended to supplement, not
replace, the advice of a trained medical professional. Consult your physician before
adopting any of the suggestions in this book, as well as about any condition that may
require diagnosis or medical attention. The author and publisher disclaim any liability
arising directly or indirectly from the use of this book.

This book is available at quantity discounts for bulk purchases.
For information, please call 1-800-289-0963.

To those who truly don't get enough protein, the beautiful children of Haiti. *Ou toujou nan kè mwen ak lapriye'm. Mwen p'ap janm bliye ou.* You are always in my heart and in my prayers. I will never forget you.

Acknowledgments

Special thanks to Joey for the use of his kitchen, to Sibella and Tim for keeping me full of coffee and homemade hummus, and to Tom for his patience and awe-inspiring hair.

Contents

Introduction

Imagine learning to swim without a pool or a coach. Or changing religions without going to church. You need the proper tools to learn new skills, and it's always helpful to have an expert there to show you the ropes every step of the way. This book is the next best thing to someone doing it for you, or having your own personal chef and nutritionist. In fact, this planner is much more convenient than having your own personal chef or nutritionist, as it can be by your side or in your kitchen twenty-four hours a day, and you don't have to pay it health insurance!

Assuming you don't have a personal chef, going vegan requires learning a bit about nutrition (something most people know very little about!), food labeling, learning to cook differently, or perhaps even learning to cook for the first time and changing your shopping habits at the grocery store. On top of all this, you'll be adjusting your daily schedule for a while as you get used to preparing more home-cooked meals. Each of these individually would be a challenge, but when going vegan, you need to acquire all these skills and make all these changes at once!

The goal of this book is to help you become a healthy and happy vegan, not just for the twelve weeks outlined here, but for as long as you want. By the time you're done following this twelve-week vegan meal plan, being vegan will be so easy that you'll barely even have to think about it. It will have become second nature. You'll learn how to cook simple, healthy vegan recipes that will keep you nourished, excited, and committed to a vegan diet. People around you may worry that you're not getting enough protein, but thanks to the well-balanced meals you'll follow, you'll know with complete confidence that you're getting more than enough protein (and exactly how much that is), and all the rest of your nutrients, too.

But perhaps you went vegan for animal rights or just because you lost a bet and don't really give a hoot about your own health. Even though they might be in the minority these days, there are certainly plenty of "junk food vegans" who love their soda, hydrogenated oils, and snack cakes and wouldn't touch a veggie unless it was deep fried. If this is what you envision for yourself in the long run, relax. No one is going to tell you that you need to be a health nut, just that you should eat some tofu along with all those potato chips, especially as a new vegan. Even if your end goal is animal rights and not longevity and wellness, you should still take the time to learn a thing or two about vegan nutrition, and plan on eating well-balanced meals (at least some of the time!) as a new vegan.

As you follow along with the planner, you'll also learn one thing that others around you might never have guessed: Going vegan is actually *fun*! You'll try new foods each week, and begin exploring new restaurants and probably new grocery stores and neighborhoods, too. Who knows, you might even meet some interesting new friends shopping the vegan section of your local health-food store! By the end of these twelve weeks, you'll be familiar with a wide variety of vegan foods and cooking techniques, and you'll be able to prepare healthy, tasty, and well-balanced meals with confidence. In fact, you'll be knowledgeable and confident enough that you'll be able to help out new vegans who feel completely overwhelmed, just like you might feel now.

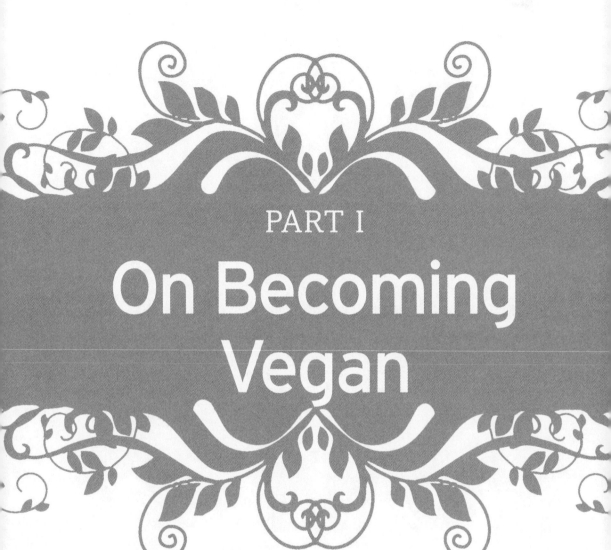

PART I

On Becoming Vegan

CHAPTER 1

On Becoming Vegan

So You've Decided You Want to Go Vegan. Now What?

Anthropologist Margaret Mead once said, "It is easier to change a man's religion than it is to change his diet." Two, three, or even more times every single day, we eat. As one of life's basic necessities, it can't be avoided. We may eat for sustenance, for pleasure, out of boredom or mindlessness, or even due to social pressure. At thirty years old, the average adult has eaten more than 30,000 meals in their lifetime. No wonder it's so difficult to make changes!

Although you're cutting all animal products (and possibly foods that may have used animals in their production) from your diet, you really won't miss a thing. As a vegan, a nearly infinite myriad of grains, herbs, fruits, vegetables, beans, and legumes from around the world is at your fingertips. There's no need to ever ask, "What do vegans eat?" It's simpler to question what vegans *don't* eat, as the list is much shorter! You may find it easiest to spend some weeks eating a vegetarian diet while gradually omitting eggs, dairy, and other animal products. Others prefer going "cold turkey." There's no right or wrong way to go vegan, but you'll need a little help along the way. If you're used to eating lots of take-out meals and processed foods, you may be wondering what's left. Going vegan will be a big change.

But if you're used to home-cooked meals made from whole ingredients and already enjoy a variety of ethnic foods, you may find the transition a little easier.

Wherever you're coming from, this book will be your mentor at every step. But first, why is the vegan diet and lifestyle so important?

Why Vegan?

If you've bought this book already, or are flipping through it at a bookstore, chances are you've already put some thought into why you want to change your diet (and your life!) by going vegan. But before you even start trying to figure out what's for dinner tonight, take a moment to think about your goals. Why do you want to go vegan? What is your personal motivation? Animal welfare? Environmentalism? Personal health?

Concerns over animal suffering may intuitively lead to a vegetarian diet, but the suffering and killing of animals in dairy and egg production inspires many well-intentioned vegetarians who learn of such practices to quickly go vegan.

Gone are the days of Old MacDonald's happily mooing dairy cows and clucking chickens. Today's cows are relentlessly milked by machines, not cheery, freckle-faced men in overalls, and chickens rarely roam free in the fresh country air. Eggs today come from hens that are tightly packed into filthy cages, stacked floor to ceiling in huge warehouses. Under these circumstances, deaths from dehydration and suffocation are common. To avoid pecking conflicts, baby chicks have their beaks sliced off at birth. Dairy-producing cows must be kept constantly pregnant in order to lactate and produce milk, which is sucked out of them by nightmarish machines, and their offspring are regularly sold to slaughterhouses as veal calves.

Such are the lives of animals used for industrialized food production. Not a pleasant life. It's no wonder that more and more people are refusing to support these practices, voting with their stomachs and pocketbooks in favor of tofu scramble over eggs from tortured hens.

Modern food production is no friend to local environments, either, as anyone who has lived near a large death factory can tell you. Neighbors of industrialized farms are constantly complaining of the air and water pollution caused by the concentrated waste of these poor animals. And the larger global environment suffers, as well. Everyone from environmental groups to the United Nations agrees that animal agriculture is one of the single largest contributors to global warming and environmental devastation. Because exponentially more water, energy, land, and resources are needed to raise and feed animals than to support a plant-based diet, one simply can't call themselves an environmentalist while still consuming animal products.

But even if compassion for animal suffering or environmental concerns just aren't your thing, personal health is a strong motivator for many people who are eating vegan. Many people of all ages report having more energy, enjoying clearer skin, and needing less sleep when following a healthy, plant-based vegan diet. Changing your diet can decrease your blood pressure in less than two months. Cholesterol lowers even more dramatically. A vegan diet is naturally cholesterol-free and is almost guaranteed to lower your cholesterol, often in as little as two weeks. But this is just the tip of the iceberg.

From significantly reduced rates of hypertension, arterial hardening, stroke, Type 2 diabetes, obesity, heart disease, and several types of cancer (prostate and breast cancer being the most well-documented), eating vegan helps prevent the vast majority of life-threatening diseases that plague modernity. Medical research and the American Dietetic Association affirm that a plant-based diet prevents many ailments, helps reverse some, and eases the symptoms of others. Veganism isn't a bulletproof vest in protecting against these killers, but it just may be the best bet.

Vegan Health and Nutrition

Of course, you do need to eat a relatively healthy diet in order to reap these benefits. After all, French fries and potato chips are animal-free, but that doesn't make them nutritious. When it comes to vegan nutrition, variety is key.

On a healthy vegan diet, you'll likely find that your intake of essential nutrients actually increases, rather than decreases, but it's still a good idea to make sure you're getting enough zinc, calcium, iron, and protein, especially as a new vegan still learning the ropes. Green, leafy vegetables are a great source of zinc and calcium. The USDA recommends an intake of three cups a week, and the menu plans in this book include greens such as spinach, collards, bok choy, and broccoli regularly. As for iron—tofu, lentils, chickpeas, tahini, and once again, those dark, leafy greens, such as spinach and kale, are reliable vegan sources.

Despite a national obsession with protein, the truth is, most Americans eat much more than recommended, and deficiency in vegans is rare. Severe protein deficiency, called *kwashiorkor*, is a very serious problem sadly endemic in developing nations such as Haiti and parts of Africa, particularly among growing children. But it's virtually unseen in developed Western countries, even among vegans.

Most vegans meet their daily requirement of protein with ease. Just a half cup of tofu, for example, contains twenty grams of protein, which is nearly half the USDA daily recommended amount for women. As a vegan, most of your protein will come from tofu, meat substitutes, beans, and lentils, but whole grains, brown rice, nut butters, soy milk, and once again, those dark, leafy greens also provide protein. Quinoa, in particular, is the queen of whole grains when it comes to protein, with sixteen grams per cup, cooked. Even as a new vegan, you don't really need to worry, as you'll probably consume more than enough protein without even thinking about it, but, as with other nutrients, make sure you're obtaining protein from more than one type of food and not just from beans or tofu alone, for example. In the words of the American Dietetic Association, "Plant sources of protein alone can provide adequate amounts of the essential and nonessential amino acids, assuming that dietary protein sources from plants are reasonably varied."

More important to be aware of is vitamin B_{12}, as it cannot reliably be obtained from vegan foods. Deficiencies of this important nutrient are admittedly rare, but long-term vegans and pregnant and breast-feeding women, in particular, need a reliable source. Because the body needs very little B_{12} and it can be stored for years, some people claim an extra supplement is not needed or suggest that omnivores are more likely to be deficient in a variety of nutrients, and the B_{12} issue for vegans is grossly overblown. While this last argument may be true, the bottom line, according to most experts, is that when it comes to B_{12}, it's best for long-term vegans to take a supplement. Better safe than sorry. Many of the recipes in this book include a vegan food supplement called nutritional yeast, which is fortified with B_{12}, as are many soy milk and veggie burger brands, so you may want to include these foods in your diet regularly.

Shopping for Vegan Foods

Health-food stores and gourmet grocers stock plenty of vegan specialty goods, but these days, even most regular chain supermarkets carry mock meats and dairy substitutes. Some stores have a separate "natural foods" aisle, while others stock the veggie burgers with the other frozen foods. Most health-food stores and co-ops are happy to place special orders, so don't be afraid to ask if there's something you'd like them to carry. Take a leisurely walk up and down each aisle of your grocery store and look at the variety of foods that you've never tried before. Chances are, many of them are vegan! The ethnic food section hides a wonderful array of vegan foods. You can usually find tahini, curry pastes, sauces, and several kinds of quick-cooking noodles. Take a careful look at the frozen foods aisle, and you're likely to find much more than just frozen veggie burgers. Frozen convenience foods may not be the healthiest option, but they're great in a pinch. Keep an eye out for vegan pot stickers, Indian meals, and bean burritos. Even if you prefer cooking most of your meals fresh, just knowing that they're available if you need them can be comforting. They'll come in handy sooner or later.

Seek out ethnic and import grocers for hidden vegan treasures, and if you're lucky, for basics at about a third the cost of other places. Miso, tempeh, and tofu, for example, are a bargain at Asian grocery stores. Besides just the deals, it's worth the extra trip to an Asian grocery to browse the mind-boggling options of exotic mock meat products you'll find there, from mock duck to vegetarian "shrimps" and "scallops." Kosher groceries stock enough dairy substitutes to fill a vegan's dreams, and Middle Eastern and Mexican grocers supply a bounty of unusual ingredients, sauces, and spices.

Experimenting with all these new foods and flavors is part of the fun of going vegan, but of course, each time you buy a new product, you'll have to take a close look to make sure that it's actually vegan. Getting in the habit of reading the ingredients list and nutritional data on the foods you buy may seem like a chore at first, but soon you'll be glad you did. Take a quick skim for the obvious animal ingredients—eggs, dairy, casein, lard—and, as someone trying to improve their health, you may want to avoid a few other things, as well. High-fructose corn syrup, for example, certainly doesn't belong in the myriad of foods into which it's added these days, such as breads and salad dressings. It's better to leave the high-fructose corn syrup and all the highly processed and packaged foods it's in on the shelf, along with monosodium glutamate (MSG), even though these are both technically vegan. Partially hydrogenated oils can be found in quite a few vegan foods, particularly in vegan dairy substitute products. While these oils are certainly tasty, many people prefer to avoid them, as well, and there are plenty of vegan margarines and cheeses that are free of these fats.

You may be concerned that all this grocery shopping for new ingredients will really add up and break the bank, but the truth is that the foundation of a healthy vegan diet is based on some of the cheapest foods on the planet. Have you seen the price of cheese lately? It's not cheap! Sure, you need to buy a few spices to get started, but with a little planning and bulk shopping, in the long run, you're more likely to see your grocery bill go down, rather than up. As a new vegan, it's helpful if you don't have to worry about prices too much in the beginning, but even if you do, you should still come out ahead.

Beans are fairly affordable when canned, but they're a bargain when prepared fresh. Lentils are even cheaper and easier to cook than dried beans. Whole grains purchased in bulk are usually less than a couple of dollars a pound, and cornmeal for making polenta is even less. In fact, the only things on a vegan diet that may be a bit more expensive are dairy- and meat-substitute products and prepared meals. If you're on a budget, opt for cheaper meat substitutes, such as TVP and homemade seitan and tofu dishes rather than store-bought seitan, and use dairy substitutes sparingly. Stretch more expensive meals or ingredients by adding a can of beans or tomatoes to whatever you're preparing, and serve with an inexpensive filler, such as rice. While not necessarily full of nutrients, pasta and rice noodles are also a bargain. Knowing the price and shopping around can help, if you've got options. For example, fresh greens may be a bargain at your local farmer's market, while apples are cheaper at your regular supermarket.

Going Vegan: Where to Start?

Common advice when going vegan is to eliminate red meats followed by white meats, and then spend some time eating just fish or a vegetarian diet before eliminating eggs, dairy, and other trace ingredients. While this method intuitively seems like a good idea and indeed works for some people, it's also a little bit backward. Here's why. Dairy, and cheese in particular, is often the most difficult food to eliminate from your diet. This is a good argument for gradually eliminating it *first* rather than last, as it may take the longest to wean you off of it. In fact, according to Dr. Neal Barnard, author of *Breaking the Food Seduction,* cheese is quite literally addictive and acts on the brain much like other drugs with a mild opiate-like effect. No wonder it's so hard to give up! The less you eat these addicting foods, the less you want them, so reducing your cheese consumption *now* is a great first step toward veganism, even if you're not already vegetarian.

If you've decided that you're motivated and disciplined enough to go "cold turkey" (or you just don't really care for milk and meat anyway), here's another piece of unconventional wisdom: Celebrate and indulge one last time. For example, if fettuccine Alfredo is one of your favorite indulgent meals, enjoy it one last time, perhaps with a glass of your favorite wine, or even on a special day—a holiday, birthday, graduation, or anniversary, and enjoy your meal guilt-free. Just make sure there aren't any leftovers around if you're going vegan the next day! Ten years down the road, you'll remember that special meal with fondness, as you happily eat your vegan dairy-free fettuccine Alfredo.

While quitting animal products cold turkey or doing a gradual elimination are both great transition methods, there is also a third way of going vegan that balances the two with a "middle path."

The "middle path" way to veganism recommends reducing your overall meat and dairy consumption while increasing consumption of plant-based foods. Think of this as a "pre-vegan" adjustment period. Take meat away from the center of your plate and put it on the side. Instead of a full steak, cook up a vegetarian stir-fry with lots of vegetables and a bit of beef over whole grains. Making a pepperoni pizza? Use half the amount of pepperoni you'd normally use, and pile on extra veggies. Don't give anything up completely, unless you're ready. Just reduce the quantity and portions of meat and dairy foods you eat while increasing your plant-based ingredients.

During this pre-vegan phase, eliminate or reduce whatever's easiest for you first, and you're not likely to miss it while you work on eliminating the other foods. For example, switch to soy or almond milk instead of dairy when cooking and baking and use vegan mayonnaise on sandwiches. You'll barely even notice both of these changes, even if you're not quite ready to make the leap from turkey sandwiches to Tofurkey slices. These are great steps to take in the week or two before you begin the meal plans set forth in this book. As an added bonus, during a pre-vegan adjustment period, you're unlikely to be faced with any of the awkward social pressures that can be associated with trying new diets, since you'll be eating relatively normal meals. You'll just be able to enjoy the process.

Making the Leap

Whatever method you choose for going vegan, gradual elimination, cold turkey, or the middle path, there's no need to leave behind your favorite foods. Whatever it is that you love, whether it's greasy pizza covered in pepperoni, cheesy pasta dishes, or just a plain old grilled burger and fries, there's a way to make it vegan. When the same sauces and spices are used in preparation, just about anything can be a pretty good stand-in for meat, and the textures and flavors of most dairy dishes are easily replicated. To experiment with ways of making your favorite meals vegan, check the index of a few good vegan cookbooks, or try typing your favorite food into an online search engine along with the words *vegan* and *recipe*. You just might be in for a surprise along with a few mouthwatering photos!

While you're easing yourself into your new vegan lifestyle, you'll need to experiment not just with new foods, but also with cooking more often at home and changing the selections you make when eating out. Use your pre-vegan time as a great excuse to have fun trying new restaurants and new vegan—or even mostly vegan—dishes. In other words, quite literally, give yourself a taste of what's to come. Ask yourself if you can really taste the cheese on your vegetarian sub sandwich piled high with veggies, and ponder just how much you would miss it.

Once you're comfortable with a slightly adjusted diet, it's time to take the next step of an honest effort at eliminating animal foods altogether. But you don't have to be perfect just yet. During these first few weeks, strive for persistence and forgiveness rather than perfection. Don't be too hard on yourself, and recognize that your experience may not be the same as what you anticipated. Close your ears to anyone who says it will be easy just as much as to anyone who tells you about how hard it will be. It won't be easy, and it won't be hard: It will be an experience that you will get through to the other side.

If you do break down and grab a hamburger one night, your goal is to respond with patience and persistence, no matter what your mind might be telling you. Your mind will let you excuse just about anything if you let it: "Well, it's all over, I may as well give up now," or "This is way too hard. I can't do this." Instead of taking this approach, allow yourself the slipup, recognizing

that change takes time. Be patient and compassionate with yourself. A minor slipup or two doesn't need to prevent you from being successful in the long run unless you let it. Give yourself a break and resolve to keep going. It's much better to eat a hamburger today and keep trying than it is to give up and eat a hamburger every day! Besides, since so many people are emotional eaters, beating yourself up over a slipup may make you more stressed and frustrated, which may lead to the urge to indulge in even more comforting non-vegan foods. Of course, just about anything you crave has a vegan version, so feel free to indulge your every whim with vegan substitutes!

If you find yourself struggling, allow yourself one meal or even one day a week to eat meat and dairy. Perhaps a Saturday or Sunday evening. Knowing you can have steak on Sunday will help you stick to your seitan throughout the week, and soon you'll find you don't need that Sunday steak after all. When you do slip up, respond not with frustration and self-loathing, but with cognizance and mindfulness. Ask yourself how you felt physically and emotionally after eating whatever it was. Did it satisfy you? Was it really what you wanted? Keeping your food log will help you identify these things and remember them for the next time you find yourself tempted. You have the rest of your life to eat vegan, and today is just one day!

When tempted, return to your original reasons for going vegan. Was it a video you saw online? Rewatch that video once or twice a week to keep it fresh in your mind. Surround yourself with reminders of your motivation, whether it's pictures of happy, rescued farm animals or pictures of pristine rainforests threatened with destruction for cattle-grazing land. It's this motivation that will keep you successful on a vegan diet.

Cravings and Changes: Be Prepared!

Although it's much easier to stick with a vegan diet than just about any other way of eating, a small minority of people who are used to eating a heavier, meatier diet may find that they are struggling with hunger as a new vegan. Remember, veganism is not a calorie-restricting diet, so the solution, of course, is simple. If you are hungry, it means you aren't getting enough calories. Eat more! It's unlikely that you'll experience this, but if you do find yourself constantly hungry or losing too much weight, opt for heavier foods, such as nuts, avocadoes, and meat substitutes, and fill up on fiber to help you feel full. Beans, lentils, and whole grains are a good source. Vegan foods tend to be lower in calories than non-vegan foods, which means you may need to eat larger meals than you may be accustomed to. For example, three ounces of lean cooked beef has more than 150 calories, while three ounces of tofu has only 60 calories. You could eat two servings of tofu and still be consuming less calories than the beef! If you're hungry, fill up your plate with more food.

Even though there's no reason to ever go hungry on a vegan diet, you may find yourself longing for specific foods. What's the difference between hunger and a food craving? If you're truly hungry, you'll eat just about anything to fill that physical void. But when you're craving a particular food, you're not actually hungry, but are usually trying to fill an emotional void with a particular comforting taste. The easiest way to distinguish between the two is to ask yourself: "Would I want to eat an apple right now? Or a green salad?" If the answer is yes, then you're probably genuinely hungry. But if the answer is no, because all you really want is some ice cream or chocolate, then you're experiencing a food craving.

Cravings are a normal part of life, no matter what diet you follow! Dealing with them as a vegan may be as simple as finding a vegan substitute for whatever it is you're craving, or it may mean getting a bit creative. Go ahead and indulge in some vegan junk food from time to time, if that's really what you need in order to keep you on the healthy path in the long run. Ice cream, potato chips, cookies, and chocolate all have vegan versions that are readily available. Just make sure it's an occasional indulgence and not a daily habit.

Even though a craving may seem to be for a particular food, it may actually be for a particular flavor or texture. A craving for sweet and sour chicken, for example, is mostly about the tangy sauce rather than the chicken itself. Why not cook up a chicken substitute or even tofu or tempeh in the same familiar sauce? Vegan substitutes can be more satisfying than you might think. Taste works in combination with all of the other senses. The visual presentation, texture, and feel of the food in our mouth, the smell, and even the sound a food makes as we chew it changes how we perceive it to taste. This is why it's so easy for vegan foods to substitute for the real thing. Take tofu scramble, for example. A good vegan scramble has tofu that is crumbled to resemble scrambled eggs, and it also has a bit of yellow coloring added to it with turmeric, curry powder, or nutritional yeast. Some recipes even call for black salt, which gives it an "eggy" smell. All of these elements fool your brain into thinking it's eating eggs while being perfectly satisfied with tofu. So go ahead, try a few substitutes with an open mind, and make your transition just a little bit easier.

Fighting cravings is also possible. Some people find that chewing gum helps a craving pass. Another tip is to eat something completely different to get your mind off whatever it is. Craving salty cheese crackers? Eat some sweet fruit. Your mind will switch gears, forget about the salt, and start enjoying the sweetness.

One of the best ways to prevent those pesky cravings is to stay hydrated. It's common knowledge that staying hydrated has a multitude of benefits for your health, and one of these benefits is to keep you feeling full. If you're feeling hungry yet you've eaten sufficient calories, it may not be food your body needs, but water. But how to make sure you've had enough? Though some nutritionists disagree that we all need eight ounces, eight times a day, this golden standard is a good goal when changing your diet and trying to increase your health.

Bring a water bottle with you wherever you go and keep it filled up. If it means buying a new purse big enough to hold your water bottle, do it! Keep a water bottle in the car, at your desk, and in your bedroom. Get in the habit of drinking a large glass of water first thing in the morning. It'll help wake you up and get your digestive system moving in the right direction to start the day. Just guzzle it down—no sipping! If you also drink a glass of water before each meal and snack, you're well on your way to meeting your hydration needs. Another idea is to fill up a pitcher of water with two quarts (a little less than two liters) of water and make sure that you drink it all throughout the day. If you're not used to drinking so much water, you may find for the first couple days that you need to urinate more frequently, but your body will soon adjust, and you'll be rewarded with more energy, better skin, enhanced digestion, and better overall health. Record each glass of water you drink in this book to make sure you're on the right track.

As your body adjusts, you may experience a bit of bloating as a new vegan. Although it's not often talked about, there's also the possibility of a bit of extra gas. Not everyone experiences this, but it can certainly be discouraging if you do! You can prevent bloating and gas before they even happen by drinking plenty of water. If you're cooking beans from scratch, make sure they're fully cooked, and switch out the soaking water with fresh water before cooking. When using canned beans, draining and rinsing them well helps rid the beans of the sugars that produce gas. Another culprit may be too much processed meat substitutes or even too much soy milk. Try sticking to simpler meals with fewer mock meats and switching to almond milk until your body adjusts to your new diet. Ease back into the offending foods slowly, with small portions to start.

But it might not even be your diet that is causing gas! Many enthusiastic new vegans are eager to experience everything the world of vegan food has to offer and end up overeating, which can also lead to gas. Consider your portion sizes. Maybe it's just too much food for your body to digest. Avoid eating when you're not actually hungry, and try not to eat too late at night.

Too late? Already bloated or gassy? Your first plan of attack is to drink a couple of glasses of water, and after that, get moving! Even though you might feel like you're about to burst like a balloon, a bit of exercise gets everything moving through your digestive track quicker. Even just fifteen minutes of brisk walking will help calm things down.

Staying Vegan: A Long-Term Lifestyle Change

As a vegan, your entire relationship to food will change. This is why going vegan is much, much easier than losing weight! More often than not, weight-loss diets fail. Why? Because most diets rely on restricting food calories or carbohydrates, which requires mental strength and willpower that most of us just don't have. Dieters still want that chocolate cookie or fried chicken, and without the strength and willpower to resist, they give in to temptation. Going vegan is easier than any other diet not only because you don't need to restrict calories or carbohydrates but also because you don't have to rely on willpower. Weight-loss diets fail in the long term because nothing actually changes. The desire for junk foods or to overeat is still there. As a vegan, you won't want that cookie anymore, and you certainly won't want that fried chicken (and if you do, you'll choose the vegan cookie and the fried seitan). No, you don't need to somehow cultivate the iron will and self-control of a Buddhist monk to control your desires for meat and dairy. The difference is, as a vegan, your desires will change. Instead of relying on willpower, you just won't want to eat meat and dairy. So how do you get to the point where you honestly don't desire those non-vegan foods anymore?

Veganism is not just another diet. It's a long-term lifestyle change. You'll be changing not just the food on your plate, but also your mind. Don't worry; you're not going to wake up tomorrow with the sudden urge to shave your head, get a tattoo, or run away to India (well, you might, but most people don't!). But by investing the effort in exploring a vegan lifestyle, you've already begun the process of self-change. If animal cruelty is more important to you than a hamburger, then you won't want that hamburger. Because you've picked up this book to explore going vegan, your priorities and motivations have already begun to change. What you want to eat today is different from what you wanted to eat two weeks ago, and it will be different from what you want to eat two weeks from now, too. It's not just your mind that

changes, but also your physical sense of taste. This is certainly good news for new vegans!

The longer you're vegan, the easier it becomes because your taste buds will change over time. Ever noticed that the more you eat spicy foods, the more heat you can tolerate? If you've ever gone a month or more without having a sugary soda, you'll know that the first time you do, it tastes unbearably sweet! This is because your taste buds react differently and adapt to whatever it is that you feed them over time.

Whether or not you're a smoker, certain medications, and even your genetics all play a role in developing and changing your own personal sense of taste. And, whether or not you change your diet, it's natural for your sense of taste to adapt and change over time as you age, and, sadly, as your taste buds die off over time. It may take one month or it may take six, but at some point, you'll look at a pile of melting cheese and think to yourself that it looks rubbery and smells like mold—guaranteed.

But even with an array of all the best vegan ice creams, chicken wings, and hot dogs, it won't always be easy to stay vegan. Your personal support system will have a huge effect on your success. Here are a few ways to make things a little bit easier for you.

Living and Eating with Omnivores

When you tell people you're eating vegan, something magical happens, and it seems that everyone you know turns into an amateur nutritionist! Be prepared for lots and lots of questions and advice from people who are simply curious or well-intentioned yet ill advised. Everyone from your closest family to strangers on the street will want to know where you get your protein from and why you don't drink milk. Usually, they'll then start telling you how much they love cheese and how they could never go vegan. Meanwhile, if you're trying to eat, your meal is getting cold. There will be times when you're happy to chat and talk about how much you love tofu, but when you're in a hurry or just plain hungry, you'd rather eat in peace and enjoy your meal without having to defend your every bite. Offering to have the conversation later, after you've eaten, is a polite way to respond. You might also refer people to a few of your favorite books about vegan nutrition. But there's no substitute for learning as much as possible. The more you know about the ethical, environmental, and health issues behind a vegan diet, the more comfortable and confident you'll feel when engaged in conversations—willingly or not—with others.

Keep in mind that no matter who says what, you don't always need to defend yourself to those folks who are less than well-intentioned when engaging you in discussions about your diet. Taking an ethical stance is not always easy, but if you know that you are doing the right thing for yourself and for the world, then it will be just a little bit easier. Who cares what everyone else thinks?

Friends, family, and coworkers will gradually get bored of offering their opinion of your every meal, but holidays and special events can be difficult to navigate, even for people who have been vegan for years. With a little communication and planning in advance, there's no need for any social faux pas. When it comes to special meals like Thanksgiving or dinner parties, don't expect your host to accommodate you without a little effort on your part, too. It's always your responsibility to make sure your dietary needs are met. Offer to bring a vegan dish (or two or three!) to share, or, if your host would like more help,

share a few of your favorite recipes or substitution ideas. Food is always a central part of holidays and social engagements, but if the goal is to come together as friends and family, the food should be what helps—not hinders—special events.

For formal restaurant meals, try to take a look at the menu in advance whenever possible, and don't be afraid to politely ask the wait staff to help accommodate you. Unless the menu says "no substitutions," substitute away! Hold the cheese and chicken on the pasta special and ask for extra veggies. A smile and a thank-you go a long way when making special requests with wait staff or inquiring about ingredients and substitutions. If you're faced with nothing but grilled chicken and other meaty entrées on the menu, take a look at the appetizers and salads. You may be able to make a great meal out of what you find there. If there's really nothing you can eat, many chefs are happy to create a special meal upon request. Even better? Call in advance to ask about your options as a vegan and to let them know you'll be requesting a vegan meal.

Sit-down catered events are a little bit trickier, as there may be nothing on the menu to choose from. In a pinch, try to take a server aside discreetly, let them know where you're sitting, and request a plate with whatever side dishes they've got. Many are the times vegans have been relegated to eating a plain baked potato and plain steamed broccoli at weddings, fund-raisers, and corporate seminars around the country, but poking at a pile of bland veggies is much less awkward than sitting in front of an empty plate, or worse, a plate filled with food you can't even poke at.

But no matter where you're eating, either at home in your own kitchen or in a five-star restaurant, the only person who ultimately matters is you. If you're sick of telling people exactly how you get your protein every day, start asking how many grams of fiber your inquisitors get each day. Or where their vitamin K comes from! As a new vegan, you'll have enough on your plate (pardon the pun) without worrying about what everyone else is concerned about! First and foremost, take good care of yourself.

Avoid Temptation

Out of sight, out of mind is certainly a truism. If you're surrounded by bacon-cooking housemates or family, it will be more difficult for you than if you're living alone or with supportive folks who are along for the ride. If your family is willing to compromise, why not ask them if they'd help you out by not eating meat in front of you? They can grab a burger for lunch while you're at work, but come dinner, it's teriyaki tempeh time with no complaints! If your fridge is filled with tempting foods, distraction will help you out until your cravings subside. Keep yourself busy, out of the kitchen, and away from temptation! It may sound like simple advice, but try to keep your mind occupied with things other than food. Read a good magazine or browse the newspaper while sipping a soy latte at a local coffeehouse if the temptation is too great at home. Try a new yoga class to occupy your evenings, or stock up on DVDs that you've been wanting to watch.

It's a bit more difficult to control your environment outside of the home. Social situations can lead to pressure to eat just to feel normal. Until you feel comfortable as a vegan and are past temptation, consider avoiding group meals when possible. Instead of meeting up for lunch with someone who might not be supportive, meet at a café for coffee or tea. Bring a few of your own hors d'oeuvres to share at a party, so you'll be less tempted by other foods.

Another way to keep food out of sight and out of mind is to turn off the TV. It's full of advertisements for foods that are rarely healthy, much less vegan. When was the last time you saw a commercial for tofu or fresh spinach on TV? Watch your favorite shows online or record them to watch later while skipping the piles of fast-food ads.

Find a Support Network

If you don't have support within your home, find it outside the home or make your own! If you're lucky enough to have friends who are already vegan, now's the time to let them know what you're doing and ask them for advice. Even if it's just a casual acquaintance, most people who are already vegan will be happy to share their experience and a few tips with you. After all, everybody likes talking about themselves! If you don't know anyone personally, turn to your computer to find sources of virtual support. Use the Internet to help you find other vegans in your community or check the bulletin boards of your health-food store. Vegetarian organizations and environmental groups often host vegan potlucks or restaurant trips where you can get to know other vegans to mentor you along the way. Online vegetarian message boards are also filled to the brim with helpful folks from all over the world who are sure to be up at all hours of the night. Before long, you'll be the expert whom other new vegans are coming to for advice!

Educate Yourself

Whether or not you have a strong support network (but especially if you don't), educating yourself with the facts about a plant-based diet will help keep you motivated if times get tough.

Read up as much as possible about veganism and vegan health, browse vegan cookbooks for ideas, and subscribe to a vegetarian magazines or e-mail lists to keep yourself immersed in vegetarian culture. Many health-food stores offer free or low-cost vegan cooking classes. Surrounding yourself (and your online world) with constant reminders will only help you even more. Follow a few vegan bloggers on Twitter, and download vegan podcasts to listen to while you walk the dog or do the dishes.

Why You Need This Book

Time and time again, many well-meaning folks stop eating milk, eggs, and dairy and end up eating nothing but French fries, chips and salsa, or next to nothing at all, then wonder why they feel tired all the time after trying out a lifestyle that is supposed to be so healthy! They blame it on the veganism, claim they aren't getting enough protein, then switch back to eating beef and cheese, or at least fish and milk. Of course, it's not lack of protein that is getting these unhealthy vegans down, it's a complete lack of *all* nutrients. Usually they say they didn't know what to eat, or that they were hungry all the time. Once you know about the incredible amount of options that vegans have to choose from, that sounds absolutely silly, but it happens quite frequently. It's why you need this book, and it's why you need to eat well as a new vegan!

The meal plans in this book gradually introduce you to the wide variety of foods available to you on a vegan diet. You'll try simple meals such as vegetable marinara and veggie burgers, traditional favorites from around the world such as pad thai from Thailand and chana masala from India, and you'll get a taste of vegan staples such as seitan, tempeh, and dairy substitutes.

The preparation techniques and ingredients vary from day to day, so you'll never get bored with your meals, and there's always something new to try. Instead of spending time scouring your cookbook library or the Internet for vegan meal ideas, and wondering what to eat while you adjust to a vegan diet, the meal plans will do all the work for you.

While following the meal plans, you won't have to worry about nutrition, either. Besides including plenty of fresh fruits and vegetables, each day's meals are planned with attention to adequate protein, calcium, iron, and zinc, and while you may want to take a vitamin B_{12} supplement as a vegan, you'll often get more than enough from the foods included. While the USDA recommends no more than 1,500 to 2,300 milligrams of sodium per day and 36 to 63 grams of fat, you'll often consume much less than this.

Another bonus? While most Americans get about half the daily recommended fiber intake of 25 to 38 grams, you'll be getting more than 30 grams almost every single day. Increased fiber consumption has a myriad of benefits, including reduced risk of heart disease and colorectal cancer, lowered cholesterol, and regulated blood sugar.

Don't let a lack of energy due to too much soda and not enough fruit get you down. Nobody likes a cranky vegan! Eating a well-balanced diet will help keep you energized and motivated to continue eating vegan. You can eat vegan stress-free and worry-free as you follow the meal plans, as this book does all of the work for you. And if eating vegan is your goal, then you need to eat properly, particularly as a new vegan, whether you want to or not!

Of course, whole grain chips dipped in a healthy salsa with fresh tomatoes or lots of veggies is a great snack. Just as long as it's not breakfast, lunch, and dinner, too.

How to Use This Book

Each day, the meal planner provides you with simple meals that are easily adaptable to a busy lifestyle. Whether you're a single student, a working parent with a family to feed, or somewhere in between, you'll find the recipes quick enough to prepare on a daily basis. Weekend breakfasts are a bit more indulgent, and lunches are always planned with busy mornings and easy transport to the office in mind. Hopefully you have access to a fridge and a microwave or toaster oven at work, and can reheat leftovers. Nearly all of the dinner meals can be prepared in less than thirty minutes.

The menu plans rely heavily on ingredients that are easily accessible (and affordable!) to most people year-round, but similar foods can be used. For example, the suggested fruits are usually apples, pineapple, or bananas, but the most important thing is not so much that you eat a banana or an apple per se, but rather that you eat at least one piece of fresh fruit. Pineapple is a great source of vitamin C, apples are high in fiber, and bananas are very filling, but there's no reason that tangerines, watermelon, mangos, and pears can't substitute for any of these. When it comes to fruit, eat what you like. Just like the type of fruit is merely a suggestion, so is the quantity. Within reason, it's impossible to eat too much fresh raw fruits and vegetables! So eat more fresh fruit each day, and snack on extra baby carrots and snap peas, if you'd like. In fact, it's encouraged.

A word of caution, however, when selecting fresh fruits and veggies. Anything that comes in a package and needs an ingredients list doesn't count as fresh raw fruit. The same goes for veggies. Banana chips, for example, are no substitute for the real thing. Skeptical? Read the label on a bag of banana chips; you'll see that they're coated in oil, with added sugar and often added salt, as well. If you must substitute for fresh produce, go for frozen fruits and veggies over canned, which nearly always have preservatives or added sugars and salts.

Grains are fairly interchangeable in the meal plans, as well, though each type has their advantages. Quinoa is a favorite among vegans for its nutty taste and high protein content. Couscous is not technically a whole grain, so it's a bit lower in nutrients, but it cooks nearly instantly. You might prefer brown rice or white rice, as they're most familiar, and you may find that you begin to love instant rice for its convenience. If you're bored of grains, most stir-fries and curries do just as well paired with noodles.

Recipes are provided for some ingredients that you may occasionally prefer to purchase pre-made, such as hummus, vegan pesto, and salsa. When substituting these (or when making any other substitutions, for that matter), take a look at the nutritional information to make sure that the store-bought versions are of similar nutritional quality to the ones provided in this book. Keep the nutritional information of store-bought goods handy by recording it in the extra space provided in Chapter 2.

In that chapter, you'll find the list of common vegan foods helpful for making any substitutions or for adding any extra snacks to your meal plan. A few minor substitutions here and there are just fine, but you'll want to keep careful track of your nutritional intake for any larger or frequent substitutions to make sure you're getting enough nutrients.

As you gain more experience in creating vegan meals, you'll find ways to personalize basic meals. A basic hummus wrap, for example, could have grated vegan cheese, pickles, olives, or sprouts, if you like them, and a tofu scramble can always have extra mushrooms or hot sauce, or whatever veggies you need to use up. You'll be able to track these variations using Chapter 2.

Before You Start

A week or so before you begin, start to prepare your kitchen. Gradually get rid of any non-vegan foods or condiments, and start stocking up on vegan pantry items. (See Chapter 2: Vegan Staples.) Gather up a few reusable storage containers for leftovers and for transporting food and snacks with you. Even if you are at home during the day and don't need to worry about bringing lunch into the office, there will inevitably be some times during the next twelve weeks when you'll need a meal or at least some snacks when you're out and about. Having something ready to go will make your life much easier.

Get Ready . . .

The equipment and utensils needed in a vegan kitchen vary little from what any other home cook might need. A blender for making healthy fruit smoothies is essential, and a food processor is helpful for making sauces such as hummus and pesto. Rather than working up a sweat grating carrots, a food processor will do the trick in ten seconds. It's definitely worth it if you're cooking for more than just one or two people. Quality chopping knives and a cutting board are standard for any cook, as are a large skillet or sauté pan, a stockpot for soups, and some oven

basics, such as a casserole dish and a baking pan. With these few items, you'll be prepared to create almost all of the recipes in this book. Though not an essential, a rice steamer means one less pot on the stove to worry about. After adding liquid and just about any grain (not just rice), you can walk away without worry.

Get Set . . .

At the beginning of each week, take a few minutes to skim through the meal plans and make sure you understand the requirements for the days ahead.

Each day's meal plans provides three balanced meals and a healthy snack. The plans are designed with the caloric needs of the average American woman in mind and provide 1,800 calories or less each day. Most men will need to increase the portion sizes of each meal in order to meet their caloric needs, about 2,200 on average. Smaller women or those hoping to reduce weight may want to reduce their intake to about 1,600 calories per day while maintaining a total fat intake of 20 to 35 percent of total calories, and keeping protein to about 10 to 35 percent. Refer to the chart at the end of this chapter to figure out your own daily nutritional needs.

Read each recipe and check the serving size carefully. If you're cooking for more than just one, make sure you have enough food to adjust your portion sizes as needed, while still having enough leftovers as required by the meal plans.

Check to make sure you understand each ingredient and preparation instruction. Do you know where you can find each ingredient at your local grocery store? Take plenty of time on the weekend to go to the grocery store, and do enough shopping to last you through the week.

Go for Your Goals

Get ready for day one. Write your goals down for your first day eating vegan and set a timeline for your transition. Don't just think about your goals; actually *write them down.* Just the simple act of writing switches on the gears in your brain, preparing you to go from thought into action. Effective goals take a bit of thought and effort. They should be as specific and concrete as possible, with an actionable timeline. They should also be quantifiable, so that you can assess your progress. "Eat healthier" or even "go vegan" are not specific time-oriented goals. Define your intentions clearly, using positive statements. Rather than "I won't eat eggs and cheese," try "Starting tomorrow, I will eat a plant-based diet every day for twelve weeks. I will keep a food log every day, and spend fifteen minutes at the end of every week reviewing my progress." If you've decided to transition more slowly, be as specific as possible with your goals. Instead of "I will eat mostly vegan for two months and then go fully vegan on January 1st," define your boundaries concretely. What does "mostly vegan" mean to you? Perhaps your goal is to eat two vegan meals a day, or to eat vegan Monday through Friday for two months. Be as specific as possible and keep your goals handy. Check in with them at least once a week to monitor your progress.

Have you written down your goals? Good. Let's continue.

Some people find it helpful to make visual representations of their goals to keep handy to constantly remind themselves and focus their mind on the target. This can be as simple as a picture of a happy pig (or an unhappy cow connected to a milking machine) taped to your refrigerator or framed next to your bed, or as comprehensive as a photo collage set on your computer desktop. While many New Age psychologists believe that having such a "vision board" allows your subconscious mind to actively work at making your visions become reality, you don't have to buy into any metaphysics to know that having pictures around will keep your conscious mind focused on your goals.

Are you ready yet for day one as a vegan?

Just one more thing.

Have you selected when day one is going to be? Pick your day, whether it's tomorrow or still a month away, and commit to it. Take the steps you need to be fully prepared by the time day one rolls around. Be confident that by the time you get to day one, you'll be ready. For convenience in using this planner, make day one a Monday, and spend the Sunday before getting ready for the coming week.

Using the Meal Planner: Daily Logging

It's human nature to notice and remember the negative things while underemphasizing the positives. But by logging and journaling your meals, you'll remember both equally. Feeling down on day twenty-one? Review your notes from a previous day when you were feeling fantastic. That amazing feeling of clarity will come back again soon. But the most important reason to log your meals is because *it works.*

In a now-famous study of American dieters by Kaiser Permanente, researchers discovered one simple key to dietary change. All things being equal to a control group, people were more able to control their eating habits and lost more weight when they simply wrote down what they ate every day. Just the act of tracking their food intake alone made people more consciously aware of what (and how much!) they were eating. The weight loss was marked. The journaling group lost twice as much weight as their nonjournaling peers. When it comes to veganism, weight loss and caloric intake may not be the focus, but the tools are the same for changing your diet successfully. Journaling keeps you accountable to yourself and increases your mindfulness and awareness. How many times a week do you really eat cheese anyway? If you're at all like most people, chances are you haven't got a clue.

As you progress through the days, be diligent and honest about recording your meals and snacks. This planner provides daily journaling space for you to note the food you've eaten, its nutrition (calories, fat, carbohydrates, fiber, and protein), how many servings you had, and when you ate the food. You may find it helpful to note where you ate, or with whom, as well as any substitutions you made in food choices or food preparation. If you substituted an orange for a handful of carrots or used peanut oil instead of olive oil while cooking a meal, make sure that you list it even if it seems like it wouldn't make much of a difference. This will not only help jog your memory about a particular meal later on, but it can also help you identify even more eating patterns. Do you tend to overeat or be tempted more when you're alone or with others? Is it always while watching TV late at night that you find yourself craving sweet desserts?

Take a few moments to note how you feel periodically each day, or after a meal. Did a fruit smoothie make you feel wide awake and energized at the beginning of the day, or was it not filling enough, leaving you hungry by 10 A.M.? Some people find that too many mock meats feel heavy in their stomach and make them sluggish while other people like the satisfying "fullness" of a denser meal. Write these things down in the section titled "Thoughts About Today" so you can begin to see any emerging patterns to help you understand what's right for you. Make sure you also note any slipups. If you find yourself scarfing down some cheese, write it down in this journaling section and note what else was going on with you that day to help figure out why you went for that cheese. Perhaps what you were really craving was salt, not salty cheese, and a bit of chips and salsa would have sufficed. Or perhaps you didn't get enough calories that day, and you were just looking for something to fill you up quick.

At the end of each week, review your feelings and your food choices in the weekly review section of the planner. What have you learned? What was the best or easiest part of the week and what did you find the most challenging? This journaling space gives you the opportunity to not only explore your feelings about the week and any challenges you faced, but also allows you to record your favorite memories and discoveries and new foods you'd like to try. Don't forget to celebrate and note your successes, too. If you particularly loved a meal or a recipe, make a note. If you notice your skin getting remarkably clearer during Week 2, write it down, so you can remember it during Week 3 when you're experiencing temptation. If you try something new and particularly love it, write it down, and be proud of yourself! Keep a list of things to get excited about, such as vegan recipes you can't wait to try or restaurants you find that have great vegan options.

Vegan Menu Planning

By following the menus set forth in this book, you'll be sure to obtain a wide variety of nutrients, foods, and exciting meals every day, with enough variety to keep the food interesting and to keep you engaged. There'll always be something new every week. But what about when you're ready to try making a few meal plans of your own?

Each page in the daily journal includes a nutritional pyramid that you can use to take a look at the foods you're eating on a daily basis. Please note, however, that the pyramid should only be used as a visual guideline, and your daily nutritional requirements may not always match up perfectly to the pyramid's building blocks. Use this pyramid to watch how your diet fills in the food pyramids over a period of time and use this info as a springboard for more independent (but always healthy!) choices and variations over time.

Vegan meal-planning centers around combing three basic ingredients: a grain or carbohydrate, a fruit or vegetable, and a protein. That doesn't mean you can't have a meal with more than one of each, or some meals with only two, but it's a convenient way to think about creating well-balanced vegan meals. A simple vegetable stir-fry with tofu (protein) and brown rice (grain) would suit this plan perfectly, as would a bowl of whole grain cereal with soy milk (protein) and bananas.

Another way to plan healthy meals is to think of foods in fours, instead of threes. The Physicians Committee for Responsible Medicine (PCRM) divides healthy vegan foods into four equal categories: fruits, vegetables, legumes, and grains. The nutritionists at PCRM suggest that a day of vegan meals should be portioned relatively equally between these foods. If you can't easily identify which of these four groups a food belongs to, chances are it's been heavily processed and is a food you should be eating minimally.

Whichever way works best for you, whether in threes or fours, plan to get a wide variety within each food group. Broccoli is wonderfully nutritious, but you'll need to eat more vegetables than just broccoli in order to maintain a healthy and well-rounded diet. If you ate broccoli on Monday, try cauliflower on Tuesday and green beans on Wednesday. Similarly, don't rely on just one

source of protein, but eat a variety of nuts, beans and legumes, and lentils throughout the day and throughout the week.

Need a convenient way to remember to vary your veggies? Remember this: *eat the rainbow*. Think of the colors of each fruit and vegetable—red strawberries, orange bell peppers, yellow squash, green romaine, blue blueberries, and purple eggplant—and try to incorporate each color from time to time. It may be oversimplifying what nutritionists surely spent years studying, but "eat the rainbow" is an easy way to remember that each color found in nature provides a different nutrient, and for a healthy variety of nutrients, a mishmash of colors is best.

Every day should include at least one serving of fresh, raw fruits or vegetables, such as raw veggies dipped in hummus or dressing, a green salad, or even just an apple. Obviously, the more fresh, raw, uncooked fruits and veggies you can include regularly, the better, and most days you'll easily get several servings rather than just one. But on busy days or when getting into new habits, it's easy to forget. Habitually eating fresh fruit first thing in the morning or making fruit the first snack you reach for is a good way to make you get something fresh every day. At the end of the day, ask yourself if you've had at least one serving of fresh, raw produce that day.

No matter what else you're eating, include several servings of green, leafy vegetables a week for optimum nutrition. There's just no substitute for fresh, raw, leafy greens, which are the most nutrient-dense foods on the planet. And finally, because it bears repeating, when planning your own vegan menus, don't forget that a healthy vegan diet requires a reliable source of vitamin B_{12}, preferably more than one.

Welcome to the wonderful world of veganism! You're going to love it!

Nutritional Guidelines

Recommended Daily Intake	
Calories	1,800*
Fat	36g–63 g
Protein	18g–63 g
Sodium	1,500 mg–2,300 mg
Fiber	25 g–38 g
Carbohydrates	135 g–200 g
Sugar	<12 g added sugar
Zinc	8 mg–11 mg
Calcium	1,000 mg–1,200 mg
Iron	8 mg–18 mg
Vitamin D	13.5 mcg
Vitamin B12	2.4 mcg

*To better personalize these values, calculate your recommended daily calorie intake based on your weight. If you are female, multiply your weight by 11. If you are male, multiply your weight by 12. Intakes for fat, protein, and carbohydrates should increase or decrease proportionally. All other values should stay the same. Consult a trusted health professional to ensure your personal goals are as accurate and healthy as possible.

CHAPTER 2

Vegan Pantry

Vegan Staples

Use this list as a guideline to help keep your cupboard and pantry well-stocked, so that you always have the ingredients needed to whip up a quick and healthy meal, whether it's breakfast, lunch, or dinner.

Perishables

You shouldn't have to buy onions, garlic, and potatoes more than once a month.

- Fresh fruit
- Garlic
- Hummus
- Onions
- Potatoes
- Tofu
- Veggies for snacking: snow peas, baby carrots, broccoli florets

Freezer Goods

- Frozen fruit for smoothies
- Frozen veggies
- Veggie burgers (or other meat substitutes)
- Ice for smoothies

Refrigerated Staples and Other Condiments

Most of these items are used in small quantities, so a one-time purchase will last for months.

- Balsamic vinegar
- Barbecue sauce
- Dijon mustard
- Ketchup
- Maple syrup
- Olive oil
- Peanut butter (or other nut butters for variety—soy nut butter or almond butter are common)
- Salad dressings
- Sesame oil
- Soy milk (buy in aseptic boxes)
- Soy sauce
- Tahini
- Vegan mayonnaise
- Vegan margarine

Cupboard Staples

Invest in a collection of mason jars for easy storage.

- Breakfast cereal
- Cocoa powder
- Couscous

- Egg substitute
- Flour
- Lentils
- Noodles
- Nutritional yeast
- Oatmeal or other whole grain cereal mix
- Pasta
- Quinoa (or other whole grains)
- White rice or brown rice

Breads

If you're usually just cooking for one, these items will fare better and last longer in the freezer.

- Bagels
- Flour or corn tortillas
- Pita bread
- Whole grain bread

Convenient Canned Goods

Stock up on a few extra "heat and eat" canned goods, such as soup or chili, for when you don't have time to cook (or just can't be bothered).

- Canned beans (black beans, chickpeas)
- Canned soups
- Canned tomatoes
- Vegetable broth (powdered or vegetarian bouillon)
- Vegetarian baked beans
- Vegetarian chili

Spices

- Basil
- Bay leaves
- Black pepper (whole in a grinder is best)
- Cayenne pepper
- Chili powder
- Cumin
- Curry powder

- Garlic powder
- Onion powder
- Oregano
- Paprika
- Parsley
- Red pepper flakes
- Sea salt or kosher salt

Handy Snacks to Have on Hand

These are mostly optional, but you'll need something around when the mood strikes.

- Nuts
- Granola
- Dried fruit
- Popcorn
- Soy yogurt

Green Salad Fixings

Keeping a selection of salad ingredients (and dressings) on hand means you have no excuses not to get your greens!

- Artichoke hearts
- Bell peppers
- Canned corn
- Cranberries
- Croutons
- Cucumbers
- Kidney beans
- Lettuce greens (romaine, baby spinach, rocket, mixed greens)
- Sunflower seeds
- Tomatoes
- Vegetarian bacon bits

Vegan Substitution Chart

Once you know a thing or two about some common vegan substitutes, veganizing your favorite recipes is easy. With a little know-how, you can find a reasonable stand-in for just about any ingredient you need, and you can make the same cookies, cakes, and muffins you've always enjoyed with egg and dairy substitutes. Though it may seem a bit odd at first to try dairy-free dairy products, these substitutes will soon be second nature to you, and you'll rarely be able to taste the difference. In fact, since most substitutes are lower in calories and fat and are occasionally cheaper, you'll wonder why you didn't make the switch sooner! Most larger grocery stores stock several vegan substitute products, but for greater variety, stop by any natural foods store.

Vegan Substitution Chart

Instead of this:	Use this:	Notes:
Butter	Vegan margarine, soy margarine	Vegan margarine works just fine in baked goods, sauces, and just about everything. One popular brand is Earth Balance.
Milk	Soy milk, almond milk, or rice milk	Rice milk is thinner and sweeter, with less fat. Stick with soy or almond for savory dishes and baking. Rice milk works best in smoothies and with breakfast cereals.
Cream	Soy cream, coconut cream	
Parmesan cheese	Nutritional yeast, or Parmesan cheese substitute (try Parma brand)	
Egg	Store-bought egg replacer (try Ener-G or Bob's Red Mill brand), 1 T. flaxmeal mixed with 3 T. water, ¼ c. applesauce	These egg substitutes work great in baked goods such as cookies, muffins, and cakes.
Mayonnaise	Store-bought vegan mayonnaise, homemade vegan mayonnaise, hummus or pesto	Vegan mayonnaise is quite tasty, but try expanding your horizons on sandwiches with different spreads, whether homemade or store-bought.
Buttermilk	1 T. lemon juice or vinegar mixed with 1 c. unsweetened soy milk	It's not quite as thick, but the acidity of the lemon juice or vinegar provides tanginess similar to buttermilk.
Cheese	Nondairy vegan cheese made from soy, rice, or almonds	Vegan Gourmet, Daiya, and Teese are the most popular brands, but there are several on the market to choose from. Watch out for casein (milk protein) in other brands. Alternatives exist for everything from mozzarella to feta.
Chocolate	Vegan chocolate	Many chocolate bars and chocolate chips are dairy-free. Just skim the ingredients list, or look for brands labeled as vegan.
Yogurt	Soy yogurt	Try Silk or WholeSoy brand. Check the dairy section of your grocery store.
Fish sauce	Soy sauce with a squeeze of lime	A common ingredient in Thai cuisine, vegetarian fish sauce is also available at some Asian grocers.
Oyster Sauce	Vegetarian oyster sauce	Another ingredient common in Asian meals, the vegetarian version is made from mushrooms and is standard in ethnic food aisles.
Honey	Agave nectar	Agave has a similar taste and consistency to honey, making it the perfect substitute.
Meat-based stocks, chicken broth	Vegetable broth, vegetarian bouillon	Watch out for monosodium glutamate (MSG) in bouillon and powdered vegetable broth.

Nutritional Information for 250 Common Vegan Foods

Wondering what else you can eat as a vegan? Here are 250 common foods that you can safely include in a vegan diet. Though it never hurts to check the label of processed foods, all of the foods included here are free of animal additives. This list will come in handy at the grocery store when you're wondering what to eat, and when making substitutions or additions to the meal plans. You can also use this list when planning your own well-balanced vegan meals in the future.

Skim the list to find a few foods you already enjoy that are high in calcium, iron, and zinc, and make a note to include these nutrient-rich foods in your diet regularly. Use the extra space provided to note the nutritional data for store-bought foods or specific brands that you eat regularly.

Beverages

Food	Serving Size	Calories	Fat	Protein	Sodium	Fiber	Carbohydrates	Sugar	Zinc	Calcium	Iron	Vitamin D	Vitamin B12
Carrot juice	1 c.	94	0.35 g	2.2 g	68 mg	1.9 g	22 g	9.2 g	0.42 mg	57 mg	1.1 mg	0 mcg	0 mcg
Coconut water	1 c.	45	0.53 g	2.4 g	250 mg	2.4 g	9.5 g	7.1 g	0 mg	57 mg	0 mg	0 mcg	0 mcg
Coffee	8 fl oz.	5	0 g	0 g	5.3 mg	0 g	1.3 g	0 g	0 mg	5.3 mg	0 mg	0 mcg	0 mcg
Cranberry juice	1 c.	144	0 g	0 g	5 mg	0.3 g	36 g	4 g	0 mg	8 mg	0.4 mg	0 mcg	0 mcg
Grapefruit juice	1 c.	95	0.27 g	2.4 g	2.4 mg	0 g	22 g	22 g	0 mg	22 mg	0 mg	0 mcg	0 mcg
Lemonade	1 c.	99	0 g	0 g	7 mg	0.2 g	26 g	0 g	0 mg	7 mg	0.4 mg	0 mcg	0 mcg
Orange juice	1 c.	110	0 g	2 g	0 mg	26 g	22 g	0 g	350 mg	0g	0 g	0.408 mg	
Prune juice	½ c.	91	0 g	0.78 g	5.1 mg	1.3 g	22 g	21 g	0.27 mg	15 mg	1.5 mg	0 mcg	0 mcg
Tea, green	1 c.	3	0 g	0 g	2.7 mg	0 g	0 g	0 g	0 mg	0 mg	0.13 mg	0 mcg	0 mcg
Tea, black	1 c.	2	0 g	0 g	0 mg	0 g	0.71 g	0 g	0.024 mg	0 mg	0.024 mg	0 mcg	0 mcg
Tomato juice (no added salt)	1 c.	41	0.1 g	1.8 g	24.3 mg	1 g	10.3 g	8.6 g	0.4 mg	24.3 mg	1.0 mg	0 IU	0 mcg
Water	1 c.	0	0 g	0 g	0 mg	0 g	0 g	0 g	0 mg	0 mg	0 mg	0 mcg	0 mcg

Dairy Replacements

Food	Serving Size	Calories	Fat	Protein	Sodium	Fiber	Carbohydrates	Sugar	Zinc	Calcium	Iron	Vitamin D	Vitamin B₁₂
Apple butter	2 T.	40	0 g	0 g	0 mg	2 g	8 g	8 g	0 mg	1.9 mg	0 mg	0 mcg	0 mcg
Almond milk, sweetened	1 c.	60	2.5 g	1 g	150 mg	1 g	8 g	7 g	1.5 mg	450 mg	0.7 mg	100 IU	3 mcg
Almond milk, unsweetened	1 c.	40	4 g	1 g	180 mg	1 g	2 g	0 g	0 g	450 mg	4%	0 g	0 g
Rice milk	1 c.	120	2 g	0.4 g	86 mg	0 g	24 g	0 g	0 mg	20 mg	0.2 mg	0 mcg	0 mcg
Soy hot chocolate	1 c.	100	2 g	6 g	95 mg	1 g	20 g	15 g	4%	300 mg	6%	30%	50%
Soy milk	1 c.	90	4.5 g	7 g	29 mg	2 g	5 g	1 g	0 mg	80 mg	1.4 mg	3 mcg	0.36 mg
Soy milk, chocolate	1 c.	120	2.5 g	5 g	140 mg	3 g	19 g	16 g	0.6 mg	300 mg	1.08 mg	0 IU	3 mcg
Soy yogurt	1 c.	140	2.5 g	5 g	20 mg	0.5 g	28 g	19 g	0 mg	8 mg	0 mg	0 IU	0 mcg
Tofu crumbles	¼ block	178	12 g	15 g	2 mg	1 g	5 g	0 g	2 mg	421 mg	3 mg	0 mcg	0 mcg
Vegan cheese	1 slice	40	2 g	1 g	120 mg	0 g	5 g	0 g	0 mg	200 mg	0 mg	0 IU	0 mcg
Vegan cream cheese	2 T.	90	8 g	2 g	115 mg	2 g	3 g	1 g	0 mg	20 mg	0.36 mg	0 IU	0 mcg
Vegan sour cream	2 T.	28	1.9 g	3 g	85 mg	0 g	<1 g	0 g	0 mg	0 mg	0 mg	0 IU	0 mcg

Fruits

Food	Serving Size	Calories	Fat	Protein	Sodium	Fiber	Carbohydrates	Sugar	Zinc	Calcium	Iron	Vitamin D	Vitamin B₁₂
Apple	1 small	77.5	0.3 g	0.4 g	1.5 mg	3.6 g	20.6 g	15.5 g	0.1 mg	8.9 mg	0.2 mg	0 IU	0 mcg
Apricots	1 c., halved	74.4	0.6 g	2.2 g	1.6 mg	3.1 g	17.4 g	14.3 g	0.3 mg	20.2 mg	0.6 mg	0 mcg	0 mcg
Avocado	1 oz.	44.8	4.1 g	0.6 g	2 mg	2 g	2.4 g	0.2 g	0.2 mg	3.4 mg	0.2 mg	0 IU	0 mcg
Banana	1 small	89.9	0.3 g	1.1 g	1 mg	2.6 g	23.1 g	12.4 g	0.2 mg	5.1 mg	0.3 mg	0 IU	0 mcg
Blackberries	1 c.	62	0.64 g	1.4 g	1.4 mg	7.2 g	14 g	7.2 g	1.4 mg	42 mg	1.4 mg	0 mcg	0 mcg
Blueberries	1 c.	84.4	0.5 g	1.1 g	1.5 mg	3.6 g	21.4 g	14.7 g	0.2 mg	8.9 mg	0.4 mg	0 IU	0 mcg
Cantaloupe melon	1 c., balls	60.2	0.3 g	1.5 g	28.3 mg	1.6 g	15.6 g	13.9 g	0.3 mg	15.9 mg	0.4 mg	0 mcg	0 mcg
Cherries	1 c.	86.9	0.3 g	1.5 g	0 mg	2.9 g	22.1 g	17.7 g	0.1 mg	17.9 mg	0.5 mg	0 mcg	0 mcg
Coconut	½ c.	136	13 g	1.2 g	7.7 mg	3.5 g	5.8 g	2.3 g	0.38 mg	5.4 mg	0.77 mg	0 mcg	0 mcg
Cranberries	1 oz.	86.2	0.4 g	0 g	0.8 mg	1.6 g	23.1 g	18.2 g	0 mg	2.8 mg	0.1 mg	0 mcg	0 mcg
Currants	1 c.	63	0.25 g	1.1 g	1.1 mg	4.5 g	16 g	7.9 g	0 mg	37 mg	1.1 mg	0 mcg	0 mcg
Dates	1 date	66.5	0 g	0.4 g	0.2 mg	1.6 g	18 g	16 g	0.1 mg	15.4 mg	0.2 mg	0 IU	0 mcg
Figs	1 fruit	46	0.21 g	0.63 g	0.63 mg	1.9 g	12 g	10 g	0 mg	22 mg	0 mg	0 mcg	0 mcg
Grapes	1 c.	61	0.3 g	0.91 g	1.8 mg	0.91 g	15 g	15 g	0 mg	13 mg	0 mg	0 mcg	0 mcg
Grapefruit	1 large	107	0.37 g	3.3 g	0 mg	3.3 g	27 g	23 g	0 mg	40 mg	0 mg	0 mcg	0 mcg
Honeydew melon	1 c.	64	0.2 g	1.8 g	32 mg	1.8 g	16 g	14 g	0 mg	11 mg	0 mg	0 mcg	0 mcg
Kiwi	1 fruit	55	0.91 g	0.91 g	2.7 mg	2.7 g	14 g	8.2 g	0 mg	31 mg	0 mg	0 mcg	0 mcg
Kumquats	4 fruits	54	0.75 g	1.5 g	7.5 mg	5.3 g	12 g	6.8 g	0 mg	47 mg	0.75 mg	0 mcg	0 mcg
Lemon	1 lemon	11.7	0 g	0.2 g	0.5 mg	0.2 g	4.1 g	1.1 g	0 mg	3.3 mg	0 mg	0 mcg	0 mcg
Lime	1 lime	11	0 g	0.2 g	0.9 mg	0.2 g	3.7 g	0.7 g	0 mg	6.2 mg	0 mg	0 mcg	0 mcg
Mango	1 c.	107	0.36 g	1.6 g	3.3 mg	3.3 g	28 g	25 g	0 mg	16 mg	0 mg	0 mcg	0 mcg
Oranges	1 large	87	0.21 g	1.9 g	0 mg	3.7 g	22 g	17 g	0 mg	74 mg	0 mg	0 mcg	0 mcg
Passion fruit	1 fruit	17.5	0.1 g	0.4 g	5 mg	1.9 g	4.2 g	2 g	0 mg	2.2 mg	0.3 mg	0 mcg	0 mcg
Peaches	1 fruit	61	0.35 g	1.6 g	0 mg	3.1 g	16 g	13 g	0 mg	9.4 mg	0 mg	0 mcg	0 mcg
Pears	1 fruit	121	0.23 g	0 g	2.1 mg	6.3 g	31 g	21 g	0 mg	19 mg	0 mg	0 mcg	0 mcg
Pineapple	1 c.	82.5	0.2 g	0.9 g	1.7 mg	2.3 g	21.6 g	16.3 g	0.2 mg	21.5 mg	0.5	0 IU	0 mcg
Plums	1 fruit	31	0.22 g	0.67 g	0 mg	0.67 g	7.3 g	6.7 g	0 mg	4 mg	0 mg	0 mcg	0 mcg
Pomegranate	1 fruit	105	0.51 g	1.5 g	4.6 mg	1.5 g	26 g	26 g	0 mg	4.6 mg	0 mg	0 mcg	0 mcg
Raspberries	1 c.	64	1.2 g	1.2 g	1.2 mg	8.6 g	15 g	4.9 g	0 mg	31 mg	1.2 mg	0 mcg	0 mcg
Strawberries	1 c.	48.6	0.5 g	1 g	1.5 mg	3 g	11.7 g	7.4 g	0.2 mg	24.3 mg	0.6 mg	0 IU	0 mcg
Tangerine	1 c.	103	0.6 g	1.6 g	3.9 mg	3.5 g	26 g	20.6 g	0.1 mg	72.2 mg	0.3 mg	0 mcg	0 mcg
Watermelon	1 c.	46	0.17 g	1.5 g	1.5 mg	0 g	12 g	9.2 g	0 mg	11 mg	0 mg	0 mcg	0 mcg

Grains

Food	Serving Size	Calories	Fat	Protein	Sodium	Fiber	Carbohydrates	Sugar	Zinc	Calcium	Iron	Vitamin D	Vitamin B₁₂
Amaranth	¼ c.	182	3.2 g	7 g	10 mg	4.5 g	32 g	0 g	1.5 mg	75 mg	3.7 mg	0 mg	0 mg
Bagel	1 bagel (3" diameter)	146	0.9 g	5.7 g	255 mg	1.3 g	29 g	2.9 g	1.1 mg	50.7 mg	3.4 mg	0 mcg	0 mcg
Barley, flakes	1 c.	141	1.1 g	4 g	186 mg	3.4 g	32 g	6.8 g	1.6 mg	15 mg	11 mg	27 mcg	2 mg
Barley, pearled	¼ c.	176	0.56 g	5 g	4.5 mg	8 g	39 g	0.5 g	1 mg	15 mg	1.5 mg	0 mcg	0 mg
Bulgur	1 c.	151	0.4 g	5.5 g	9.1 mg	9.1 g	35 g	0 g	1.8 mg	18 mg	1.8 mg	0 mcg	0 mcg
Buckwheat flour	¼ c.	101	0.9 g	3.9 g	3.3 mg	3 g	21 g	0.9 g	0.9 mg	12 mg	1.2 mg	0 mcg	0 mcg
Buckwheat groats	1 c.	155	1 g	5.7 g	6.7 mg	4.5 g	34 g	1.5 g	1 mg	12 mg	1.3 mg	0 mcg	0 mcg
Cornmeal	½ c.	251	1.4 g	5.5 g	2.1 mg	4.8 g	53 g	0.68 g	0.68 mg	3.4 mg	2.7 mg	0 mcg	0 mcg
Couscous	1 c., cooked	175	0.17 g	6.3 g	7.8 mg	1.6 g	36 g	0 g	0 mg	13mg	0 mg	0 mcg	0 mcg
Couscous, whole wheat	¼ c.	173	1.5 g	7.5 g	0 mg	4.5 g	36 g	0.8 g	0 mg	20 mg	1.82 mg	0 mcg	0 mcg
Cream of wheat	1 c.	31.5	0.6 g	4.4 g	364 mg	1.4 g	31.5 g	0.2 g	0.4 mg	154 mg	12 mg	0 mcg	0 mcg
English muffin	1 muffin	140	1.1 g	5.4 g	248 mg	1.5 g	27.4 g	1.8 g	0.7 mg	102 mg	2.4 mg	0 mcg	0 mcg
Flour tortilla	1 tortilla (51 grams)	146	3.1	4.4 g	249 mg	0 g	25.3 g	0 g	0 mg	97.4 mg	1 mg	0 mcg	0 mcg
Granola	⅓ c.	194	10 g	5.2 g	71.1 mg	3.7 g	23.2 g	7.7 g	1.2 mg	36.7 mg	1.4 mg	0 mcg	0 mcg
Grits	1 c.	143	0.5 g	3.4 g	540 mg	0.7 g	31.1 g	0.2 g	0.2 mg	7.3 mg	1.5 mg	0 mcg	0 mcg
Millet	¼ c.	189	2 g	5.5 g	2.5 mg	4.5 g	37 g	0 g	1 mg	4 mg	1.5 mg	0 mcg	0 mcg
Oat bran	¼ c.	56	2 g	4 g	1 mg	3 g	15 g	0 g	1 mg	13 mg	1 mg	0 mg	0 mg
Oat groats	¼ c.	110	2.5 g	7 g	0 mg	4 g	27 g	1 g	0 mg	20 mg	0 mg	0 mcg	0 mcg
Oats, steel-cut	½ c.	152	2.7 g	6.6 g	0.78mg	4.3 g	26 g	0 g	1.6 mg	21 mg	2 mg	0 mg	0 mg
Pita	1 pita (6½" diameter)	165	0.7 g	5.5 g	322 mg	1.3 g	33.4 g	0.8 g	0.5 mg	51.6 mg	1.6 mg	0 mcg	0 mcg
Polenta	½ c.	252	1.1 g	6 g	2.1 mg	5 g	54 g	0.44 g	0.5 mg	3.4 mg	2.8 mg	0 mcg	0 mcg
Quinoa	1 c.	222	3.6 g	8.1 g	13 mg	5.2 g	39.4 g	0 g	2 mg	31.5 mg	2.8 mg	0 mcg	0 mcg
Rice, brown	1 c.	216	1.8 g	5 g	9.8 mg	3.5 g	44.8 g	0.7 g	1.2 mg	19.5 mg	0.8 mg	0 mcg	0 mcg
Rice cake	1 oz.	110	1.2 g	2 g	19.9 mg	1.2 g	22.7 g	0.2 g	0.8 mg	3.1 mg	0.4 mg	0 mcg	0 mcg
Rice noodles	1 c.	192	0.4 g	1.6 g	33.4 mg	1.8 g	43.8 g	0 g	0.4 mg	7 mg	0.2 mg	0 mcg	0 mcg
Rice, white	1 c.	169	0.3 g	3.5 g	8.7 mg	1.7 g	36.7 g	0.1 g	0.7 mg	3.5 mg	0.2 mg	0 mcg	0 mcg
Rye	¼ c.	146	1.3 g	6.4 g	2.5 mg	6.4 g	30 g	0.42 g	1.7 mg	14 mg	1.3 mg	0 mcg	0 mcg
Spelt	1 c. cooked	246	1.6 g	10 g	9.7 mg	7.6 g	51 g	0 g	2.4 mg	19.4 mg	3.2 mg	0 mcg	0 mcg
Spelt bread	1 slice	70	0 g	3 g	150 mg	2 g	16 g	2 g	0 mg	0 mg	0 mg	0 mcg	0 mcg
Soba noodles	1 c.	113	0.1 g	5.8 g	68.4 mg	0 g	24.4 g	0 g	0.1 mg	4.6 mg	0.5 mg	0 mcg	0 mcg

Grains

Food	Serving Size	Calories	Fat	Protein	Sodium	Fiber	Carbohydrates	Sugar	Zinc	Calcium	Iron	Vitamin D	Vitamin B12
Taco shell, hard	1 shell (5" diameter)	58.2	2.6 g	0.9 g	48.6 mg	0.6 g	7.9 g	0.2 g	0.2 mg	12.6 mg	0.2 mg	0 mcg	0 mcg
Teff	½ c. uncooked	354	2.3 g	12.8 g	11.5 mg	7.7 g	70 g	1.8 g	3.5 mg	173 mg	7 mg	0 mcg	0 mcg
Triticale	¼ c.	161	1 g	6.3 g	2.4 mg	0 g	35 g	0 g	1.7 mg	18 mg	1.2 mg	0 mcg	0 mcg
Pan-fried polenta	1 oz.	101	1 g	2.3 g	9.8 mg	2 g	21.5 g	0.2 g	0.5 mg	1.7 mg	1 mg	0 mcg	0 mcg
Pizza dough	2 oz.	120	1.1 g	4 g	240 mg	2 g	24 g	0 g	0 mg	0 mg	0 mg	0 mcg	0 mcg
Popcorn	1 c.	30.6	0.3 g	1 g	0.3 mg	1.2 g	6.2 g	0 g	0.3 mg	0.8 mg	0.2 mg	0 mcg	0 mcg
Vegetable pasta	½ c.	76	0.57 g	2.9 g	3.4 mg	0 g	14 g	0 g	0.57 mg	10 mg	0.57 mg	0 mcg	0 mcg
Wheat berries	½ c.	151	1 g	6 g	0 mg	4 g	29 g	0 g	5.6 mg	15 mg	7 mg	0 mcg	0 mcg
Whole grain bread	1 slice	69.1	1.1 g	3.5 g	110 mg	1.9 g	11.3 g	1.7 g	0.4 mg	26.6 mg	0.7 mg	0 mcg	0 mcg
Whole grain cereal	¾ c.	100	0.5 g	2 g	190 mg	2.7 g	23.2 g	5 g	15 mg	1000 mg	18 mg	39.9 mcg	6 mcg
Whole wheat pasta	½ c.	100	1.7 g	5 g	308 mg	2.5 g	23 g	0 g	0.5 mg	14 mg	1.5 mg	0 mcg	0 mcg

Meat Replacements

Food	Serving Size	Calories	Fat	Protein	Sodium	Fiber	Carbohydrates	Sugar	Zinc	Calcium	Iron	Vitamin D	Vitamin B12
Black bean burger	1 burger	264	1 g	15 g	391 mg	9.7 g	49 g	1.4 g	2.6 mg	79 mg	3.8 mg	0 mcg	0 mcg
Falafel	1 patty	57	3 g	2.3 g	50 mg	1 g	5.4 g	0 g	0.26 mg	9.2 mg	0.58 mg	0 mcg	0 mcg
Ground beef substitute (sautéed)	½ c.	60	0.5 g	13 g	270 mg	3 g	6 g	0 g	0 mg	60 mg	1.8 mg	0 IU	0 mcg
Seitan	3 oz.	90	1 g	18 g	380 mg	1 g	3 g	0 g	0 mg	0 mg	1 mg	0 IU	0 mcg
Tempeh	½ c.	161	9.2 g	16 g	7.5 mg	0 g	7.5 g	0 g	0.83 mg	93 mg	2.5 mg	0 mcg	0 mcg
Tofu, baked	½ c.	88.2	5.3 g	10.3 g	15.1 mg	1.1 g	2.1 g	0.8 g	1 mg	253 mg	2 mg	0 IU	0 mcg
Vegetarian chicken	3 oz.	120	5 g	9 g	210 mg	4 g	11 g	0 g	0 mg	35 mg	15 mg	0 IU	0 mcg
Vegetarian chicken patty burger	1 patty	140	5 g	8 g	590 mg	2 g	16 g	1 g	0 mg	0 mg	0 mg	0 IU	0 mcg
Veggie burger	1 patty	124	4.4 g	11 g	398 mg	3.4 g	10 g	0.7 g	0.9 mg	95.2 mg	1.7 mg	0 mcg	1.4 mcg
Vegan sausage	1 patty	80	3 g	10 g	260 mg	1 g	3 g	1 g	0 mg	3 mg	1.44 mg	0 IU	2.1 mcg
Vegetarian pepperoni	13 slices	50	1 g	9 g	240 mg	1 g	2 g	0 g	0 mg	0 mg	0.36 mg	0 mcg	0 mcg
Vegetarian hot dogs	1 link	80	2 g	11 g	390 mg	3 g	5 g	0 g	0 mg	2 mg	4 mg	0 mcg	0 mg

Nuts and Seeds

Food	Serving Size	Calories	Fat	Protein	Sodium	Fiber	Carbohydrates	Sugar	Zinc	Calcium	Iron	Vitamin D	Vitamin B12
Almond	1 oz.	161	13.8 g	5.9 g	0.3 mg	3.4 g	6.1 g	1.1 g	0.9 mg	73.9 mg	1 mg	0 IU	0 mcg
Brazil nuts	¼ c.	218	22 g	4.75 g	1 mg	2.5 g	4 g	0.77 g	1.35 mg	53.25 mg	0.8 mg	0 mcg	0 mcg
Cashew	1 oz.	155	12.3 g	5.1 g	3.4 mg	0.9 g	9.2 g	1.7 g	1.6 mg	10.4 mg	1.9 mg	0 IU	0 mcg
Chestnuts, roasted	½ c.	175	1.6 g	2.1 g	1.4 mg	3.6 g	38 g	7.9 g	0.71 mg	21 mg	0.71 mg	0 mcg	0 mcg
Chia seed	½ oz.	69	4.4 g	2.2 g	2.7 mg	5.3 g	6.2 g	0 g	0.49 mg	89 mg	0 mg	0 mcg	0 mcg
Flaxseed	2 T.	104	8.2 g	3.5 g	5.9 mg	5.3 g	5.7 g	0.39 g	0.78 mg	50 mg	1.2 mg	0 mcg	0 mcg
Hazelnut	¼ c.	180	18 g	4.3 g	0 mg	2.9 g	4.9 g	1.1 g	0.57 mg	33 mg	1.4 mg	0 mcg	0 mcg
Macadamia nuts	¼ c.	239	25 g	3 g	2 mg	3 g	5 g	2 g	0 mg	28 mg	1 mg	0 mcg	0 mcg
Nuts, mixed	1 oz.	172	15.7 g	4.3 g	85.7 mg	1.5 g	6.2 g	1.2 g	1.3 mg	29.7 mg	0.7 mg	0 IU	0 mcg
Peanuts, dry-roasted	1 oz.	164	13.9 g	6.6 g	1.7 mg	2.2 g	6 g	1.2 g	0.9 mg	15.1 mg	0.6 mg	0 mcg	0 mcg
Peanuts, oil-roasted	1 oz.	168	14.7 g	7.8 g	89.6 mg	2.6 g	4.3 g	1.2 g	0.9 mg	17.1 mg	0.4 mg	0 IU	0 mcg
Pecans	1 oz.	193	20.2 g	2.6 g	0 mg	2.7 g	3.9 g	1.1 g	1.3 mg	19.6 mg	0.7 mg	0 IU	0 mcg
Pine nuts	¼ c.	190	17 g	8.3 g	1.2 mg	1.2 g	4.8 g	0 g	0 mg	8.3 mg	3.6 mg	0 mcg	0 mcg
Pistachios	¼ c.	170	13 g	6.4 g	0.3 mg	3 g	8.5 g	2.4 g	0.61 mg	33 mg	1.2 mg	0 mcg	0 mcg
Pumpkin seeds	¼ c.	185	16 g	8.6 g	6.2 mg	1.4 g	6.2 g	0.34 g	2.4 mg	15 mg	5.1 mg	0 mcg	0 mcg
Soy nut	1 oz.	126	6.1 g	11.1 g	0.6 mg	2.3 g	9.2 g	0 g	1.3 mg	39.2 mg	1.1 mg	0 mcg	0 mcg
Sunflower seeds	¼ c.	65	5.7 g	2.6 g	0.34 mg	1.3 g	2.2 g	0.34 g	0.57 mg	13 mg	0.8 mg	0 mcg	0 mcg
Walnuts	1 oz.	185	18.4 g	4.3 g	0.6 mg	1.9 g	3.9 g	0.7 g	0.9 mg	27.7 mg	0.8 mg	0 IU	0 mcg

Spices

Food	Serving Size	Calories	Fat	Protein	Sodium	Fiber	Carbohydrates	Sugar	Zinc	Calcium	Iron	Vitamin D	Vitamin B12
Basil	¼ c.	3	0.11 g	0.32 g	0.42 mg	0.42 g	0.42 g	0 g	0.11 mg	16 mg	0.32 mg	0 mcg	0 mcg
Bay leaf	2 leaves	18	0.45 g	0.45 g	1.3 mg	1.5 g	4.3 g	0 g	0.23 mg	47 mg	2.4 mg	0 mcg	0 mcg
Cayenne pepper	1 t.	5.6	0.3 g	0.2 g	0.5 mg	0.5 g	1 g	0.2 g	0 mg	2.6 mg	0.1 mg	0 mcg	0 mcg
Caraway seed	1 T.	22	0.98 g	1.3 g	1.1 mg	2.5 g	3.3 g	0 g	0.37 mg	46 mg	1.1 mg	0 mcg	0 mcg
Chili pepper	1 pepper	18	0.2 g	0.91 g	4.1 mg	0.91 g	4.1 g	2.3 g	0 mg	6.4 mg	0.45 mg	0 mcg	0 mcg
Chives	2 T.	2	0.061 g	0.18 g	0.18 mg	0.18 g	0.24 g	0.12 g	0.061 mg	5.6 mg	0.12 mg	0 mcg	0 mcg
Cilantro	¼ c.	0.9	0 g	0.1 g	1.8 mg	0.1 g	0.1 g	0 g	0 mg	2.7 mg	0.1 mg	0 mcg	0 mcg
Clove	1 t. ground	7	0.44 g	0.13 g	5.4 mg	0.76 g	1.4 g	0 g	0.022 mg	14 mg	0.2 mg	0 mcg	0 mcg
Cinnamon	1 t.	6.2	0 g	0.1 g	0.2 mg	1.3 g	2 g	0.1 g	0 mg	25.1 mg	0.2 mg	0 mcg	0 mg
Cocoa powder	2 T.	40	1 g	2 g	0 mg	2 g	6 g	0 g	0 mg	0 mg	3.6 mg	0 mcg	0 mcg
Cumin	1 t.	7	0.43 g	0.35 g	3.3 mg	0.22 g	0.86 g	0 g	0.098 mg	18 mg	1.3 mg	0 mcg	0 mcg
Dill	¼ c. fresh	1	0.025 g	0.07 g	1.4 mg	0.045 g	0.16 g	0 g	0.023 mg	4.7 mg	0.16 mg	0 mcg	0 mcg
Fennel seed	1 T.	20	0.88 g	0.94 g	5.2 mg	2.4 g	3.1 g	0 g	0.24 mg	70 mg	1.1 mg	0 mcg	0 mcg
Garlic	1 T.	13	0.084 g	0.51 g	1.4 mg	0.17 g	2.8 g	0.084 g	0.084 mg	15 mg	0.17 mg	0 mcg	0 mcg
Ginger root	1 t.	5	0 g	0.13 g	0.81 mg	0.13 g	1.1 g	0.13 g	0 mg	1 mg	0.063 mg	0 mcg	0 mcg
Horseradish	1 T.	7	0.15 g	0.15 g	47 mg	0.45 g	1.6 g	1.2 g	0.15 mg	8.4 mg	0 mg	0 mcg	0 mcg
Lavender	1 t.	0	0 g	0 g	0 mg	0 g	1 g	0 g	0 mg	0 mg	0 mg	0 mcg	0 mcg
Marjoram	1 t. dried	2	0 g	0 g	0 mg	0 g	0 g	0 g	0 mg	11 mg	0 mg	0 mcg	0 mcg
Mint	2 T.	4.9	0.1 g	0.4 g	3.4 mg	0.8 g	0.9 g	0 g	0.1 mg	22.4 mg	1.3 mg	0 mcg	0 mcg
Mustard seeds	1 t.	18	1.1 g	0.94 g	0.19 mg	0.56 g	1.3 g	0.26 g	0.22 mg	20 mg	0.37 mg	0 mcg	0 mcg
Paprika	1 T.	21	0.93 g	1.1 g	2.4 mg	2.6 g	4 g	0.71 g	0.29 mg	13 mg	1.7 mg	0 mcg	0 mcg
Parsley	¼ c.	5	0 g	0 g	7.5 mg	0 g	1.3 g	0 g	0 mg	18 mg	1.3 mg	0 mcg	0 mcg
Peppermint	1 T.	1	0.015 g	0.06 g	0.5 mg	0.13 g	0.24 g	0 g	0.018 mg	3.9 mg	0.081 mg	0 mcg	0 mcg
Rosemary	1 T. fresh	2	0.1 g	0.05 g	0.44 mg	0.24 g	0.36 g	0 g	0.017 mg	5.4 mg	0.12 mg	0 mcg	0 mcg
Tarragon	1 t. dried	2	0.042 g	0.14 g	0.37 mg	0.042 g	0.3 g	0 g	0.024 mg	6.8 mg	0.19 mg	0 mcg	0 mcg
Thyme	1 T.	2	0 g	0.14 g	0.22 mg	0.34 g	0.58 g	0 g	0.048 mg	9.7 mg	0.41 mg	0 mcg	0 mcg
Turmeric	1 t.	8	0.22 g	0.18 g	0.84 mg	0.47 g	1.4 g	0 g	0.089 mg	4.1 mg	0.91 mg	0 mcg	0 mcg
Wasabi	1 T.	9	0.081 g	0.41 g	1.4 mg	0.65 g	1.9 g	0 g	0.16 mg	10 mg	0.081 mg	0 mcg	0 mcg

Vegetables

Food	Serving Size	Calories	Fat	Protein	Sodium	Fiber	Carbohydrates	Sugar	Zinc	Calcium	Iron	Vitamin D	Vitamin B₁₂
Alfalfa sprouts	1 c.	10	0 g	1 g	2 mg	1 g	1 g	0 g	0 mg	11 mg	0 mg	0 mcg	0 mcg
Artichokes	1 medium	60	0 g	4 g	114 mg	6.9 g	13 g	0 g	0.63 mg	56 mg	1.6 mg	0 mcg	0 mcg
Asparagus	1 c.	27	0.15 g	2.7 g	2.7 mg	2.7 g	5.3 g	2.7 g	1.3 mg	32 mg	2.7 mg	0 mcg	0 mcg
Asparagus, steamed	½ c.	19.8	0.2 g	2.2 g	12.6 mg	1.8 g	3.7 g	1.2 g	0.5 mg	20.7 mg	0.8 mg	0 mcg	0 mcg
Beans, baked	½ c.	120	0.5 g	6 g	480 mg	6 g	24 g	9 g	2.1 mg	40 mg	2.7 mg	0 IU	0 mcg
Beans, black	1 c. canned	227	0.9 g	15.2 g	1.7 mg	15 g	40.8 g	0 g	1.9 mg	46.4 mg	3.6 mg	0 IU	0 mcg
Beans, butter	½ c. canned	110	0.5 g	6 g	420 mg	5 g	19 g	0 g	0 mg	60 mg	1.79 mg	0 mcg	0 mcg
Cannellini beans	½ c. canned	154	0.44 g	9.2 g	6.6 mg	6.6 g	29 g	0 g	1.3 mg	96 mg	3.9 mg	0 mcg	0 mcg
Beans, fava	1 c. canned	182	0.57 g	13 g	375 mg	10 g	31 g	0 g	2.6 mg	67 mg	2.6 mg	0 mcg	0 mcg
Beans, garbanzo	¾ c. canned	213	2 g	9 g	534 mg	7.1 g	41 g	0 g	1.8 mg	57 mg	1.8 mg	0 mcg	0 mcg
Beans, kidney	1 c. canned, rinsed	210	2.6 g	13 g	759 mg	10 g	38 g	5.1 g	0 mg	87 mg	2.6 mg	0 mcg	0 mcg
Beans, lima	¼ c. uncooked	151	0.45	9.4 g	8 mg	8.5 g	28 g	4 g	1.3 mg	36 mg	3.6 mg	0 mcg	0 mcg
Beans, mung	¼ c. uncooked	180	0.6 g	12 g	7.8 mg	8.4 g	32 g	3.4 g	1.4 mg	68 mg	3.5 mg	0 mcg	0 mcg
Beans, navy	½ c. canned	148	0.56 g	9.9 g	586 mg	6.7 g	27 g	0.37 g	1 mg	62 mg	2.4 mg	0 mcg	0 mcg
Beans, pinto	1 c. cooked	205	2 g	12 g	23 mg	12 g	36 g	0 g	2.4 mg	102 mg	2.4 mg	0 mcg	0 mcg
Beans, refried	1 c.	217	2.8 g	12.9 g	1069 mg	12.1 g	36.3 g	1.1 g	1.5 mg	78.6 mg	4 mg	0 IU	0 mcg
Beans, yellow wax	1 c.	27	0.14 g	1.6 g	2.7 mg	1.8 g	6.1 g	1.3 g	0.39 mg	35 mg	1.2 mg	0 mcg	0 mcg
Bean sprouts	1 c.	31	0 g	3 g	0 mg	2 g	6 g	4 g	0 mg	0 mg	0 mg	0 IU	0 mcg
Beets	1 c.	58	0.3 g	2.7 g	105 mg	4.1 g	14 g	9.5 g	0 mg	22 mg	1.4 mg	0 mcg	0 mcg
Beet greens	1 c.	8	0 g	0.77 g	87 mg	1.5 g	1.5 g	0.38 g	0 mg	45 mg	1.2 mg	0 mcg	0 mcg
Bok choy	1 c.	20	0 g	2 g	90 mg	2 g	4 g	0 g	4.3 mg	32 mg	1.1 mg	0 mcg	0 mcg
Broccoli, raw	1 c.	30.9	0.3 g	2.6 g	30 mg	2.4 g	6 g	1.5 g	0.4 mg	42.8 mg	0.7 mg	0 mcg	0 mcg
Broccoli, steamed	1 stalk, 1 c.	49	0.6 g	3.3 g	57.4 mg	4.6 g	10.1 g	1.9 g	0.6 mg	56 mg	0.9 mg	0 IU	0 mcg
Broccoli rabe	1 c., chopped	8.8	0.2 g	1.3 g	13.2 mg	1.1 g	1.2 g	0.2 g	0.3 mg	43.2 mg	0.9 mg	0 mcg	0 mcg
Brussels sprouts	1 c.	61	1 g	4 g	33 mg	4 g	14 g	0 g	0 mg	56 mg	2 mg	0 mcg	0 mcg
Cabbage	1 c.	22	0.1 g	0.91 g	16 mg	1.8 g	5.5 g	3.6 g	0 mg	43 mg	0.91 mg	0 mcg	0 mcg
Cauliflower	1 c.	25	0.1 g	2 g	30 mg	2.5 g	5.3 g	2.4 g	0.3 mg	22 mg	0.4 mg	0 IU	0 mcg
Carrots	1 c.	52.5	0.3 g	1.2 g	88.3 mg	3.6 g	12.3 g	6.1 g	0.3 mg	42.2 mg	0.4 mg	0 mcg	0 mcg
Carrots, baby	3 oz.	29.8	0.1 g	0.5 g	66.3 mg	2.5 g	7 g	4 g	0.1 mg	27.2 mg	0.8 mg	0 IU	0 mcg
Cauliflower	1 c.	25	0.11 g	2 g	30 mg	3 g	5 g	2 g	0 mg	22 mg	0 mg	0 mcg	0 mcg

Vegetables

Food	Serving Size	Calories	Fat	Protein	Sodium	Fiber	Carbohydrates	Sugar	Zinc	Calcium	Iron	Vitamin D	Vitamin B₁₂
Celery	1 c.	14	0.22 g	1 g	81 mg	2 g	3 g	2 g	0 mg	40 mg	0 mg	0 mcg	0 mcg
Collard greens	1 c.	11	0.16 g	0.71 g	7.1 mg	1.4 g	2.1 g	0 g	0 mg	52 mg	0 mg	0 mcg	0 mcg
Corn on the cob	1 ear	155	3.4 g	4.5 g	29.2 mg	0 g	31.9 g	0 g	0.9 mg	4.4 mg	0.9 mg	0 IU	0 mcg
Cucumber	1 cucumber	45.1	0.3 g	2 g	6 mg	1.5 g	10.9 g	5 g	0.6 mg	48.2 mg	0.8 mg	0 IU	0 mcg
Edamame	1 c.	189	8.1 g	16.9 g	9,3 mg	8.1 g	15.8 g	3.4 g	2.1 mg	97.6 mg	3.5 mg	0 IU	0 mcg
Eggplant	1 c.	32.7	0.2 g	0.8 g	237 mg	2.5 g	8.1 g	3.2 g	0.1 mg	5.9 mg	0.2 mg	0 IU	0 mcg
Endives	2 c.	17	0.22 g	1 g	22 mg	3 g	3 g	0 g	1 mg	52 mg	1 mg	0 mcg	0 mcg
Kale	1 c.	33	0.67 g	2 g	29 mg	1.3 g	6.7 g	0 g	0 mg	90 mg	1.3 mg	0 mcg	0 mcg
Kohlrabi	1 c.	36	0.15 g	2.7 g	27 mg	5.4 g	8.1 g	4.1 g	0 mg	32 mg	0 mg	0 mcg	0 mcg
Leeks	1 c.	55	0.3 g	1.8 g	18 mg	1.8 g	13 g	3.6 g	0 mg	54 mg	1.8 mg	0 mcg	0 mcg
Lentils	¼ c. uncooked	170	0.53 g	13 g	2.9 mg	15 g	29 g	0.96 g	2.4 mg	27 mg	3.8 mg	0 mcg	0 mcg
Lettuce, iceberg	1 c.	10.1	0.1 g	0.6 g	7.2 mg	0.9 g	2.3 g	1.4 g	0.1 mg	13 mg	0.3 mg	0 IU	0 mcg
Lettuce, romaine	1 c.	8	0.1 g	0.6 g	3.8 mg	1 g	1.5 g	0.6 g	0.1 mg	15.5 mg	0.5 mg	0 IU	0 mcg
Mushrooms, portabella	1 medium	29	0.25 g	3.4 g	6.8 mg	2.3 g	5.7 g	2.3 g	1.1 mg	9.1 mg	1.1 mg	0 mcg	0 mcg
Mushrooms, shiitake	1 c.	81	0.32 g	2.9 g	5.8 mg	2.9 g	20 g	5.8 g	1.4 mg	4.3 mg	0 mg	0 mcg	0 mcg
Mushroom, white button	1 c.	16	0.24 g	2.1 g	3.6 mg	0.71 g	2.1 g	1.4 g	0.71 mg	2.1 mg	0.71 mg	0 mcg	0 mcg
Olives, green	1 oz.	40.6	4.3 g	0.3 g	436 mg	0.9 g	1.1 g	0.2 g	0 mg	14.6 mg	0.1 mg	0 IU	0 mcg
Okra	1 c.	31	0.11 g	2 g	8 mg	3 g	7 g	1 g	1 mg	81 mg	1 mg	0 mcg	0 mcg
Onion, boiled pearl	1 c.	43	0 g	0 g	0 mg	0 g	1 g	0 g	0 mg	3.1 mg	0 mg	0 mcg	0 mcg
Onion, red	1 onion	42	0 g	0 g	0 mg	0 g	1 g	0 g	0 mg	3 mg	1.2 mg	0 mcg	0 mcg
Parsnips	1 c.	100	0.44 g	1.3 g	13 mg	6.7 g	24 g	6.7 g	1.3 mg	48 mg	1.3 mg	0 mcg	0 mcg
Peas	1 c.	117	0.64 g	7.2 g	7.2 mg	7.2 g	20 g	8.7 g	1.4 mg	36 mg	1.4 mg	0 mcg	0 mcg
Peas, black-eyed	1 c. canned	199	3.8 g	6.6 g	839 mg	7.9 g	40 g	0 g	2.5 mg	41 mg	3.4 mg	0 mcg	0 mcg
Pepper, jalapeño	1 pepper	4	0.14 g	0.14 g	0.14 mg	0.42 g	0.85 g	0.42 g	0 mg	1.4 mg	0.14 mg	0 mcg	0 mcg
Pepper, green bell	1 c.	29.8	0.3 g	1.3 g	4.5 mg	2.5 g	6.9 g	3.6 g	0.2 mg	14.9 mg	0.5 mg	0 mcg	0 mcg
Pepper, roasted red bell	1 oz.	9.3	0 g	0 g	112 mg	0.9 g	3.7 g	0.9 g	0 mg	0 mg	1 mg	0 IU	0 mcg
Pepper, yellow bell	1 pepper	32	0 g	1 g	2 mg	2 g	8 g	0 g	0 mg	11 mg	1 mg	0 mcg	0 mcg
Potatoes	1 small (138 grams)	128	0.2 g	3.5 g	13.8 mg	3 g	29.2 g	1.6 g	0.5 mg	20.7 mg	1.5 mg	0 IU	0 mcg
Pumpkin	1 c.	30	0.13 g	1.2 g	1.2 mg	1.2 g	8.1 g	1.2 g	0 mg	24 mg	1.2 mg	0 mcg	0 mcg

Vegetables

Food	Serving Size	Calories	Fat	Protein	Sodium	Fiber	Carbohydrates	Sugar	Zinc	Calcium	Iron	Vitamin D	Vitamin B12
Rutabaga	1 c.	51	0.31 g	1.4 g	28 mg	4.2 g	11 g	8.5 g	0 mg	66 mg	1.4 mg	0 mcg	0 mcg
Sweet potato	1 small (60 grams)	54	0.1 g	1.2 g	21.6 mg	2 g	12.4 g	3.9 g	0.2 mg	22.8 mg	0.4 mg	0 IU	0 mcg
Spinach	1 c.	6.9	0.1 g	0.9 g	23.7 mg	0.7 g	1.1 g	0.1 g	0.2 mg	29.7 mg	0.8 mg	0 IU	0 mcg
Spinach, steamed	1 c.	41.4	0.5 g	5.3 g	126 mg	4.3 g	6.7 g	0.8 g	1.4 mg	245 mg	6.4 mg	0 IU	0 mcg
Squash, acorn	1 c.	56	0.16 g	1.4 g	4.2 mg	2.8 g	14 g	0 g	0 mg	46 mg	1.4 mg	0 mcg	0 mcg
Squash, oven-roasted butternut	1 c.	82	0.2 g	1.8 g	8.2 mg	0 g	21.5 g	4 g	0.3 mg	84 mg	1.2 mg	0 IU	0 mcg
Squash, summer	1 c.	18	0.25 g	1.1 g	2.3 mg	1.1 g	3.4 g	2.3 g	0 mg	17 mg	0 mg	0 mcg	0 mcg
Squash, spaghetti	1 c.	41.9	0.4 g	1 g	27.9 mg	2.2 g	10 g	3.9 g	0.3 mg	32.6 mg	0.5 mg	0 mcg	0 mcg
Swiss chard	1 c.	7	0 g	0.71 g	76 mg	0.71 g	1.4 g	0.36 g	0 mg	18 mg	0.71 mg	0 mcg	0 mcg
Tomato	1 medium	22.1	0.2 g	1.1 g	6.2 mg	1.5 g	4.8 g	3.2 g	0.2 mg	12.3 mg	0.3 mg	0 IU	0 mcg
Turnips	1 large	51	0.2 g	1.8 g	122 mg	3.6 g	11 g	7.3 g	0 mg	55 mg	0 mg	0 mcg	0 mcg
Water chestnuts	¼ c.	30	0 g	0.31 g	4.3 mg	0.93 g	7.4 g	1.5 g	0.31 mg	3.4 mg	0 mg	0 mcg	0 mcg
Watercress	¼ c.	1	0 g	0.17 g	3.5 mg	0 g	0.086 g	0 g	0 mg	10 mg	0 mg	0 mcg	0 mcg
Yams	1 c.	176	0.33 g	3 g	13 mg	6 g	42 g	1.5 g	0 mg	25 mg	1.5 mg	0 mcg	0 mcg
Zucchini	1 c.	19.8	0.2 g	1.5 g	12.4 mg	1.4 g	4.2 g	2.1 g	0.4 mg	18.6 mg	0.4 mg	0 mcg	0 mcg
Zucchini, sautéed	1 c.	28.8	0.1 g	1.2 g	5.4 mg	2.5 g	7.1 g	3 g	0.3 mg	23.4 mg	0.6 mg	0 IU	0 mcg

Your Favorite Foods

Food	Serving Size	Calories	Fat	Protein	Sodium	Fiber	Carbohydrates	Sugar	Zinc	Calcium	Iron	Vitamin D	Vitamin B₁₂

PART II

The Planner

WEEK 1

Congratulations! Welcome to your new adventurous life as a vegan! You've stocked your pantry, cleared out any non-vegan foods from your refrigerator, and made a date with your kitchen. This is going to be fun! Week 1 should be the easiest week, as you'll be feeling motivated and excited. We'll keep it simple this week and ease you into it with lots of familiar foods, such as spaghetti with marinara, veggie burgers, and peanut butter and jelly, as well as plenty of hearty and satisfying meals to keep you feeling full.

Don't worry too much about portion size or nutrition just yet. If you're hungry, just eat! Now is the time to focus on you and your new lifestyle. Say no to any extra personal or professional commitments that may distract you, because you need to be focused on yourself and your new diet this week. Make sure you have plenty of time in the morning to eat breakfast and pack a lunch, and save a bit of extra time in the evening to relax and enjoy the process of cooking dinner.

If your friends and family are supportive, now's the time to let everyone know what you're doing. Knowing they're watching will help keep you honest. On the other hand, if you're surrounded by naysayers, it's none of their business!

Your goal this week? Take good care of yourself, but most importantly, just eat!

Monday

Breakfast

Two slices whole grain bread, 1 T. peanut butter, 1 T. sugar-free jam, 1 banana

Cal.: 338; Fat: 10.5 g; Protein: 13.1 g; Sodium: 224 mg; Fiber: 7.4 g; Carbs.: 53.7 g; Sugar: 16.8 g; Zinc: 1 mg; Calcium: 58.3 mg; Iron: 1.7 mg; Vit. D: 0 mcg; Vit. B$_{12}$: 0 mcg

Lunch

Veggie burger with ¼ tomato, avocado, lettuce on whole grain bread, 1 c. baked beans, 1 c. orange juice

Cal.: 317.58; Fat: 10.8 g; Protein: 19.18 g; Sodium: 625.12 mg; Fiber: 10.03 g; Carbs.: 37.35 g; Sugar: 5.8 g; Zinc: 2 mg; Calcium: 161.38 mg; Iron: 3.53 mg; Vit. D: 0 mcg; Vit. B$_{12}$: 1.4 mcg

Snack

Mixed veggies (½ cucumber, 2 oz. baby carrots, ½ c. broccoli) with 3 T. hummus

Cal.: 116.92; Fat: 3.32 g; Protein: 5.38 g; Sodium: 189.5 mg; Fiber: 6.52 g; Carbs.: 19.37 g; Sugar: 6.12 g; Zinc: 1.27 mg; Calcium: 81.63 mg; Iron: 2.18 mg; Vit. D: 0 mcg; Vit. B$_{12}$: 0 mcg

Dinner

1 c. Basic Vegetable Marinara with 1 c. whole grain pasta, side green salad with 2 c. romaine lettuce, 1 tomato, and 1 diced cucumber, 2 T. Goddess Dressing

Cal.: 468.53; Fat: 18.43 g; Protein: 16.67 g; Sodium: 515.73 mg; Fiber: 16.42 g; Carbs.: 73.77 g; Sugar: 20.19 g; Zinc: 2.68 mg; Calcium: 205.83 mg; Iron: 6.15 mg; Vit. D: 0 mcg; Vit. B$_{12}$: 0 mcg

Basic Vegetable Marinara

Serves 6

4 cloves garlic
1 carrot, sliced thin
2 ribs celery, chopped
2 T. olive oil
1 (28-oz.) can diced or stewed tomatoes
1 (6-oz.) can tomato paste
1 t. oregano
1 t. parsley

2 T. chopped fresh basil
2 bay leaves
½ c. corn (optional)
½ c. sliced black olives
1 T. balsamic vinegar
½ t. crushed red pepper flakes
½ t. salt

1. Heat garlic, carrot, and celery in olive oil over medium heat, stirring frequently, for 4–5 minutes.
2. Reduce heat to medium low, then add tomatoes, tomato paste, oregano, parsley, basil, and bay leaves, stirring well to combine.
3. Cover and heat for at least 30 minutes, stirring frequently.
4. Add corn, olives, balsamic vinegar, red pepper, and salt, and simmer for another 5 minutes, uncovered.
5. Remove bay leaves before serving, and adjust seasonings to taste.

Goddess Dressing

Turn this zesty salad dressing into a dip for veggies or a sandwich spread by reducing the amount of liquids.
Yields 1½ cups

⅔ c. tahini
¼ c. apple cider vinegar
⅓ c. soy sauce
2 t. lemon juice

1 clove garlic
¾ t. sugar (optional)
⅓ c. olive oil

1. Process all the ingredients except olive oil together in a blender or food processor until blended.
2. With the blender or food processor on high speed, slowly add in the olive oil, blending for another full minute, allowing the oil to emulsify.
3. Chill in the refrigerator for at least 10 minutes before serving; dressing will thicken as it chills.

Date ____ / ____ / ____

Glasses of Water Consumed: _____

Thoughts About Today: _____

_____

_____

What I Ate Today

Time	Food Item	Amount	Calories	Fat	Carbs	Fiber	Protein
TOTAL							

Fats

Protein/Legumes

Fruits

Vegetables

Whole Grains

In a Pinch Don't have time to make marinara from scratch? Take five minutes to heat a store-bought jar on the stove and add in frozen veggies, Italian seasonings, and a bit of wine or balsamic vinegar for a fresh taste.

Tuesday

Breakfast

¾ c. whole grain cereal, 1 c. soy milk

Cal.: 223; Fat: 5.17 g; Protein: 9.67 g; Sodium: 282.33 mg; Fiber: 5.6 g; Carbs.: 35.93 g; Sugar: 7.67 g; Zinc: 20 mg; Calcium: 1413.33 mg; Iron: 25.4 mg; Vit. D: 56.2 mcg; Vit. B$_{12}$: 8.36 mcg

Lunch

Hummus (2 T.) sandwich with ½ cucumber, sprouts (½ c.), and roasted red peppers (1 oz.) on whole grain bread

Cal.: 235; Fat: 5.1 g; Protein: 11.9 g; Sodium: 448.6 mg; Fiber: 8.25 g; Carbs.: 38.9 g; Sugar: 8.8 g; Zinc: 1.7 mg; Calcium: 88.7 mg; Iron: 3.6 mg; Vit. D: 0 mcg; Vit. B$_{12}$: 0 mcg

Snack

200 calories of whole grain chips with ½ c. salsa

Record nutritional values for your choice of chips and salsa in today's journal:

Dinner

1 c. Sun-Dried Tomato Risotto with Spinach, 1 c. Caramelized Baby Carrots

Cal.: 522.67; Fat: 21.73 g; Protein: 8.8 g; Sodium: 737.33 mg; Fiber: 6.6 g; Carbs.: 71.33 g; Sugar: 25.47 g; Zinc: .56 mg; Calcium: 131.33 mg; Iron: 5.53 mg; Vit. D: 0 mcg; Vit. B$_{12}$: 4.2 mcg

---

Sun-Dried Tomato Risotto with Spinach

The tomatoes carry the flavor in this easy risotto—no butter, cheese, or wine are needed. But if you're a gourmand who keeps truffle, hazelnut, pine nut, or another gourmet oil on hand, now's the time to use it instead of the margarine. **Serves 4**

1 yellow onion, diced	1 c. fresh spinach
4 cloves garlic, minced	1 T. chopped fresh basil (optional)
2 T. olive oil	2 T. nutritional yeast (optional)
1½ c. Arborio rice	
5–6 c. vegetable broth	Salt and pepper to taste
⅔ c. rehydrated sun-dried tomatoes, sliced	

1. Heat onion and garlic in olive oil until just soft, about 2–3 minutes. Add rice, and toast for one minute, stirring constantly.
2. Add ¾ cup vegetable broth and stir to combine. When most of the liquid has been absorbed, add another ½ cup, stirring constantly. Continue adding liquid ½ cup at a time until rice is cooked, about 20 minutes.
3. Add another ½ cup broth, tomatoes, spinach, and basil, and reduce heat to low. Stir to combine well. Heat for 3–4 minutes, until tomatoes are soft and spinach is wilted.
4. Stir in nutritional yeast. Taste, then season lightly with a bit of salt and pepper. Risotto will thicken a bit as it cools.

Caramelized Baby Carrots

Baby carrots have a natural sweetness when cooked, and this recipe turns them into a treat even the pickiest veggie hater will gobble up. **Serves 4**

4 c. baby carrots	2 T. vegan margarine
Water for boiling	2 T. brown sugar
1 t. lemon juice	¼ t. sea salt

1. Simmer carrots in water until just soft, about 8–10 minutes; do not overcook. Drain and drizzle with lemon juice.
2. Heat together carrots, margarine, brown sugar, and sea salt, stirring frequently, until glaze forms and carrots are well coated, about 5 minutes.

Glasses of Water Consumed: _____

Thoughts About Today: _____

_____

_____

What I Ate Today

Time	Food Item	Amount	Calories	Fat	Carbs	Fiber	Protein
TOTAL							

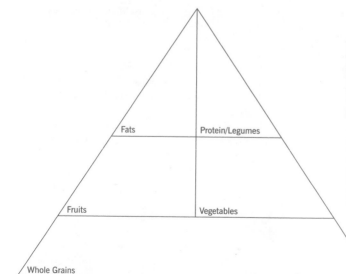

Fats

Protein/Legumes

Fruits

Vegetables

Whole Grains

Sun-Dried Tomatoes If you're using dehydrated tomatoes, rehydrate them first by covering in water for at least ten minutes, and add the soaking water to the broth. If you're using tomatoes packed in oil, add two tablespoons of the oil to risotto at the end of cooking instead of the vegan margarine.

Wednesday

Breakfast

½ c. old-fashioned oats with blueberries, almonds, and 2 t. maple syrup, 1 c. chocolate soy milk

Cal.: 530.33; Fat: 19.6 g; Protein: 18 g; Sodium: 98 mg; Fiber: 12 g; Carbs.: 83.46 g; Sugar: 40.29 g; Zinc: 2.25 mg; Calcium: 391.73 mg; Iron: 3.44 mg; Vit. D: 2.7 mcg; Vit. B$_{12}$: 3 mcg

Lunch

2 pieces Easy Vegan Pizza Bagels, 1 c. sliced strawberries, 1 c. orange juice

Cal.: 464.6; Fat: 3.5 g; Protein: 16 g; Sodium: 779.5 mg; Fiber: 8 g; Carbs.: 98.7 g; Sugar: 32.4 g; Zinc: 1.2 mg; Calcium: 390.3 mg; Iron: 4.6 mg; Vit. D: 0 mcg; Vit. B$_{12}$: .41 mcg

Snack

1 (6-inch) pita with 2 T. hummus

Cal.: 215; Fat: 3.5 g; Protein: 7.9 g; Sodium: 435.6 mg; Fiber: 3.1 g; Carbs.: 37.6 g; Sugar: .8 g; Zinc: 1.1 mg; Calcium: 63 mg; Iron: 2.4 mg; Vit. D: 0 mcg; Vit. B$_{12}$: 0 mcg

Dinner

1½ c. Black Bean and Butternut Squash Chili

Cal.: 530; Fat: 6.8 g; Protein: 29 g; Sodium: 496 mg; Fiber: 21g; Carbs.: 91 g; Sugar: 9 g; Zinc: 5 mg; Calcium: 207 mg; Iron: 7 mg; Vit. D: 0 mcg; Vit. B$_{12}$: 0mcg

---

Easy Vegan Pizza Bagels

Need a quick lunch or after-school snack for the kids? Pizza bagels to the rescue! For a real treat, shop for vegetarian "pepperoni" slices to top them off. **Serves 4**

⅓ c. pizza sauce or tomato sauce	4 bagels, sliced in half (try whole grain)
½ t. garlic powder	8 slices vegan cheese (optional)
¼ t. salt	¼ c. sliced mushrooms (optional)
½ t. basil	¼ c. sliced black olives
½ t. oregano	

1. Preheat oven to 325°F.
2. Combine pizza sauce, garlic powder, salt, basil, and oregano.
3. Spread sauce over each bagel half, and top with cheese, mushrooms, olives, or any other toppings.
4. Heat in oven for 8–10 minutes.

Black Bean and Butternut Squash Chili

Squash is an excellent addition to vegetarian chili in this Southwestern-style dish. **Serves 6**

1 onion, chopped	¾ c. water or vegetable broth
3 cloves garlic, minced	1 T. chili powder
2 T. oil	1 t. cumin
1 medium butternut squash, chopped into chunks	¼ t. cayenne pepper, or to taste
2 (15-oz.) can black beans, drained	½ t. salt
1 (28-oz.) can stewed or diced tomatoes, undrained	2 T. chopped fresh cilantro (optional)

1. In a large stockpot, sauté onion and garlic in oil until soft, about 4 minutes.
2. Reduce heat and add remaining ingredients, except cilantro.
3. Cover and simmer for 25 minutes. Uncover and simmer another 5 minutes. Top with fresh cilantro just before serving.

favourite

Day 17 vegan.

Wednesday

Glasses of Water Consumed: 5 8oz glasses (water bottles)

Thoughts About Today: Didnt plan out where I was getting what nutrients + calories from. Overate?

What I Ate Today

Time	Food Item	Amount	Calories	Fat	Carbs	Fiber	Protein
	2c. Oatmeal w/ 1cup raisins/almonds		608				
	1 bowl fruit.						
	1 bowl steamed veggies						
	handful cran/almonds						
	1 banana						
	1 corn flour tortilla						
	2 tbsp hummus						
	1/4 red bell pepper						
	1 1/2 c Chili		530	6.8g	91g	21g	29g
11:30pm	1 cup dried cran						
	1/4 cup walnuts.		185	18g			4.3g
	B12 supplement.						
TOTAL							

Fats

Protein/Legumes

Fruits

Vegetables

Whole Grains

Don't Go Without Your Joe!
You don't have to give up your daily cup-o'-joe when you go vegan! Try a soy- or coconut-milk creamer to whiten your brew, or use plain or vanilla soy milk with a bit of sugar. Most coffeehouses offer soy milk these days. If your usual neighborhood café doesn't, ask them to supply it, or find one that does.

Thursday ♡ soy free

Breakfast

12 oz. Chocolate Peanut Butter Banana Smoothie

Cal.: 288; Fat: 11 g; Protein: 10 g; Sodium: 124 mg; Fiber: 7 g; Carbs.: 45 g; Sugar: 20 g; Zinc: 1.1 mg; Calcium: 205 mg; Iron: 1.8 mg; Vit. D: 0 mg; Vit. B$_{12}$: 1.5 mg

Snack

1 c. unsweetened applesauce, 1 oz. raisins

Cal.: 186.5; Fat: 0.3 g; Protein: 1.3 g; Sodium: 8 mg; Fiber: 3.7 g; Carbs.: 49.9 g; Sugar: 39.6 g; Zinc: 0.2 mg; Calcium: 23.9 mg; Iron: 1.1 mg; Vit. D: 0 mcg; Vit. B$_{12}$: 0 mcg

Lunch

1½ c. leftover Black Bean and Butternut Squash Chili (see recipe in Week 1, Wed.), side green salad with 2 c. romaine lettuce, 1 tomato, and 1 diced cucumber, 2 T. Goddess Dressing (see recipe in Week 1, Mon.), 1 c. orange juice

Cal.: 842.2; Fat: 19.1 g; Protein: 37.5 g; Sodium: 722.2 mg; Fiber: 27.12 g; Carbs.: 138.9 g; Sugar: 40.76 g; Zinc: 6.58 mg; Calcium: 700.5 mg; Iron: 10.32 mg; Vit. D: 0 mcg; Vit. B$_{12}$: 0.41 mcg

Dinner

⅓ Green Olive and Artichoke Focaccia Pizza, 1 c. steamed cauliflower

Cal.: 246; Fat: 12.1 g; Protein: 7 g; Sodium: 859 mg; Fiber: 5.9 g; Carbs.: 32.3 g; Sugar: 5.8 g; Zinc: 1.03 mg; Calcium: 72 mg; Iron: 2.4 mg; Vit. D: 0 mcg; Vit. B$_{12}$: 0 mcg

Chocolate Peanut Butter Banana Smoothie

Yummy enough for a dessert, but healthy enough for breakfast, this smoothie is also a great protein boost after a sweaty workout at the gym. **Serves 2**

7–8 ice cubes
2 bananas
2 T. natural peanut butter
2 T. unsweetened cocoa powder
1 c. calcium-fortified soy milk

Blend together all ingredients until smooth.

(3-4 ice cubes
  1 banana
  1T natural PB.
  1T uns. cocoa powder
  1c almond milk.

Green Olive and Artichoke Focaccia Pizza

A gourmet vegan pizza with plenty of Italian seasonings; no cheese needed. **Serves 3**

1 vegan focaccia bread	¾ c. chopped artichoke hearts
1 T. olive oil	½ c. sliced mushrooms
½ t. salt	3 cloves garlic, minced
½ t. rosemary	½ t. parsley
½ t. basil	¼ t. oregano
⅓ c. tomato paste	½ t. red pepper flakes (optional)
½ c. chop sliced green olives	

1. Preheat oven to 400°F.
2. Drizzle focaccia with olive oil and sprinkle with salt, rosemary, and basil.
3. Spread a thin layer of tomato paste on the focaccia, then top with olives, artichoke hearts, mushrooms, and garlic.
4. Sprinkle with parsley, oregano, and red pepper flakes, then bake for 20 minutes, or until done.

Glasses of Water Consumed: _____

Thoughts About Today: _____

_____

_____

What I Ate Today

Time	Food Item	Amount	Calories	Fat	Carbs	Fiber	Protein
	Smoothie	12oz	288	11g	45g	7g	10g
12pm	Chili + Salad						
330p	Applesauce Snack						
TOTAL							

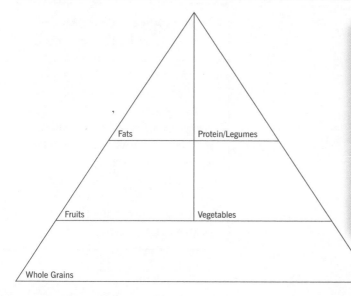

Fats

Protein/Legumes

Fruits

Vegetables

Whole Grains

What's Missing? Feeling hungry or like you're just "missing something"? It may be water that you're craving. Keep a bottle of water by your side wherever you go—in the car, in the office, in the living room—to help make sure you're getting enough. Get in the habit of guzzling a big glass of water first thing in the morning to help start your day well hydrated.

Friday

Smoothie

Breakfast

⅓ c. granola, 1 c. soy milk

Cal.: 361.5; Fat: 14.8 g; Protein: 12.6 g; Sodium: 101.6 mg; Fiber: 9.3 g; Carbs.: 48.8 g; Sugar: 24.2 g; Zinc: 1.3 mg; Calcium: 125.6 mg; Iron: 3 mg; Vit. D: 3 mcg; Vit. B$_{12}$: 0.36 mcg

Lunch

⅓ leftover Green Olive and Artichoke Focaccia Pizza (see recipe in Week 1, Thurs.), side green salad with 2 c. romaine lettuce, 1 tomato, and 1 diced cucumber, 2 T. Goddess Dressing (see recipe in Week 1, Mon.), 1 c. orange juice

Cal.: 534.2; Fat: 24.3 g; Protein: 13.5 g; Sodium: 1085.2 mg; Fiber: 9.52 g; Carbs.: 74.9 g; Sugar: 35.16 g; Zinc: 2.31 mg; Calcium: 543.5 mg; Iron: 5.32 mg; Vit. D: 0 mcg; Vit. B$_{12}$: 0.41 mcg

Snack

Mixed fruit salad with ½ apple, ½ banana, ½ c. strawberries, and ½ c. pineapple, 1 oz. cashews

Cal.: 304.25; Fat: 12.95 g; Protein: 6.8 g; Sodium: 6.25 mg; Fiber: 6.65 g; Carbs.: 47.7 g; Sugar: 27.5 g; Zinc: 1.95 mg; Calcium: 40.3 mg; Iron: 2.7 mg; Vit. D: 0 mcg; Vit. B$_{12}$: 0 mcg

Dinner

1¾ c. Italian White Bean and Fresh Herb Salad, 1 c. steamed spinach

Cal.: 349.4; Fat: 1.7 g; Protein: 20.7 g; Sodium: 195 mg; Fiber: 14.9 g; Carbs.: 65.7 g; Sugar: 1.54 g; Zinc: 2.94 mg; Calcium: 421.4 mg; Iron: 12.7 mg; Vit. D: 0 mcg; Vit. B$_{12}$: 0 mcg

Italian White Bean and Fresh Herb Salad

Don't let the simplicity of this bean salad fool you! The fresh herbs marinate the beans to flavorful perfection, so there's no need to add anything else! **Serves 4**

2 cans cannellini or great northern beans, drained and rinsed

2 ribs celery, diced

¼ c. chopped fresh parsley

¼ c. chopped fresh basil

3 T. olive oil

3 large tomatoes, chopped

½ c. sliced black olives

2 T. lemon juice

Salt and pepper to taste

¼ t. crushed red pepper flakes (optional)

1. In a large skillet, combine the beans, celery, parsley, and basil with olive oil. Heat, stirring frequently, over low heat for 3 minutes, until herbs are softened, but not cooked.
2. Remove from heat and stir in remaining ingredients, gently tossing to combine. Chill for at least one hour before serving.

Fresh Is Always Best Cans are convenient, but dried beans are cheaper, need less packaging, add a fresher flavor, and, if you plan in advance, aren't much work at all to prepare. Place your beans in a large pot, and cover with plenty of water (more than you think you'll need), then allow them to sit for at least 2 hours. Overnight is fine. Drain the soaking water and simmer in fresh water for about an hour, then you're good to go! One cup of dried beans yields about three cups cooked.

Date ____ / ____ / ____

Glasses of Water Consumed: _____

Thoughts About Today: _____

_____

_____

What I Ate Today

Time	Food Item	Amount	Calories	Fat	Carbs	Fiber	Protein
TOTAL							

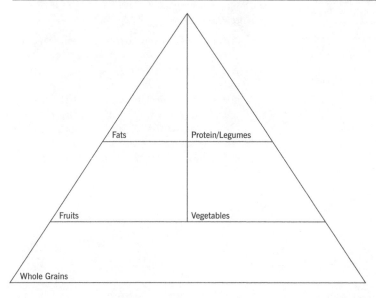

Saturday

Breakfast

1 Potato Poblano Breakfast Burrito, 1 c. orange juice

Cal.: 459; Fat: 12 g; Protein: 9.4 g; Sodium: 432 mg; Fiber: 6.4 g; Carbs.: 80 g; Sugar: 25.7 g; Zinc: 0 mg; Calcium: 408 mg; Iron: 3.1 mg; Vit. D: 0 mcg; Vit. B$_{12}$: 0.41 mcg

Lunch

Hummus wrap with ¼ c. tomatoes, ½ c. spinach, ½ c. sprouts, and 1 oz. olives in a flour tortilla, 1 c. soy milk

Cal.: 326; Fat: 13.4 g; Protein: 15.13 g; Sodium: 781.2 mg; Fiber: 5.53 g; Carbs.: 38.25 g; Sugar: 4.05 g; Zinc: 0.45 mg; Calcium: 215.63 mg; Iron: 3.38 mg; Vit. D: 3 mcg; Vit. B$_{12}$: 0.36 mcg

Snack

veggies   carrots and almonds

1 c. edamame

Cal.: 189; Fat: 8.1 g; Protein: 16.9 g; Sodium: 9.3 mg; Fiber: 8.1 g; Carbs.: 15.8 g; Sugar: 3.4 g; Zinc: 2.1 mg; Calcium: 97.6 mg; Iron: 3.5 mg; Vit. D: 0 mcg; Vit. B$_{12}$: 0 mcg

Dinner

1 c. Asian Sesame Tahini Noodles, 1 c. grilled pineapple, side green salad with 2 c. romaine lettuce, 1 tomato, and 1 diced cucumber, 2 T. Goddess Dressing (see recipe in Week 1, Mon.)

Cal.: 681; Fat: 24.5 g; Protein: 22.4 g; Sodium: 1179.9 mg; Fiber: 11.02 g; Carbs.: 108.5 g; Sugar: 26.32 g; Zinc: 4.28 mg; Calcium: 283 mg; Iron: 7.12 mg; Vit. D: 0 mcg; Vit. B$_{12}$: 0 mcg

---

Potato Poblano Breakfast Burritos

Serves 3

2 T. olive oil

2 small potatoes, diced small

2 poblano or Anaheim chiles, diced

1 t. chili powder

Salt and pepper to taste

1 tomato, diced

⅔ c. vegetarian ground beef or sausage substitute (optional)

2–3 flour tortillas, warmed

Grated vegan cheese (optional)

Ketchup or hot sauce (optional)

1. Heat olive oil in a pan and add potatoes and chiles, sautéing until potatoes are almost soft, about 6–7 minutes.
2. Add chili powder, salt and pepper, tomato, and meat substitute, and stir well to combine.
3. Continue cooking until potatoes and tomatoes are soft and meat substitute is cooked, another 4–5 minutes.
4. Wrap in warmed flour tortillas with vegan cheese and ketchup or a bit of hot sauce, if desired.

Asian Sesame Tahini Noodles

A creamy and nutty Chinese-inspired noodle dish. If you don't have Asian-style noodles on hand, spaghetti will do. **Serves 4**

1 lb Asian noodles

½ c. tahini

⅓ c. water

2 T. soy sauce

1 clove garlic

2 t. fresh ginger, minced

2 T. rice vinegar

2 t. sesame oil

1 red bell pepper, sliced thin

3 scallions, chopped

¾ c. snow peas, chopped

¼ t. crushed red pepper flakes

1. Cook noodles according to package instructions, drain well.
2. Whisk or blend together the tahini, water, soy sauce, garlic, ginger, and rice vinegar.
3. In a large skillet, heat the sesame oil, bell pepper, scallions, and snow peas for 2–3 minutes. Add tahini sauce and noodles, stirring well to combine.
4. Cook over low heat just until heated, about 2–3 minutes. Garnish with crushed red pepper flakes to taste.

Date ___ / ___ / ___

Saturday

Glasses of Water Consumed: _____

Thoughts About Today: _____

_____

_____

What I Ate Today

Time	Food Item	Amount	Calories	Fat	Carbs	Fiber	Protein
TOTAL							

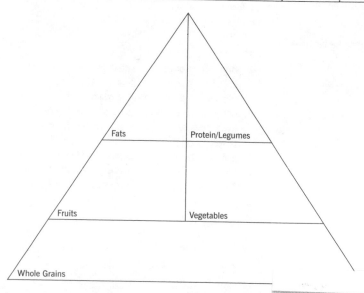

Fats

Protein/Legumes

Fruits

Vegetables

Whole Grains

Sunday

Breakfast

3 slices Easy Vegan French Toast, 1 c. strawberries, 1 c. soy milk

Cal.: 453.6; Fat: 8.6 g; Protein: 18 g; Sodium: 458.5 mg; Fiber: 13 g; Carbs.: 79.7 g; Sugar: 29.4 g; Zinc: 1.6 mg; Calcium: 242.6 mg; Iron: 4.9 mg; Vit. D: 3 mcg; Vit. B$_{12}$: 0.79 mcg

Snack

cran + almonds

1 c. soy yogurt with ⅓ c. granola, 1 c. orange juice

Cal.: 444; Fat: 12.5g; Protein: 12.2 g; Sodium: 91.1 mg; Fiber: 4.2 g; Carbs.: 77.2 g; Sugar: 48.7 g; Zinc: 1.2 mg; Calcium: 394.7 mg; Iron: 1.4 mg; Vit. D: 0 mcg; Vit. B$_{12}$: 0.41 mcg

Lunch

1 c. vegetarian baked beans on 2 slices toasted whole grain bread, 1 c. pineapple, 1 small apple

Cal.: 349.1; Fat: 2.1 g; Protein: 10.8 g; Sodium: 592.8 mg; Fiber: 13.8 g; Carbs.: 77.5 g; Sugar: 42.5 g; Zinc: 2.8 mg; Calcium: 97 mg; Iron: 4.1 mg; Vit. D: 0 mcg; Vit. B$_{12}$: 0 mcg

Dinner

1½ c. Bell Peppers Stuffed with Couscous, ½ c. black beans, 1 c. steamed broccoli

Cal.: 424.5; Fat: 8.05 g; Protein: 18.5 g; Sodium: 107.25 mg; Fiber: 16.8 g; Carbs.: 70.5 g; Sugar: 3.9 g; Zinc: 1.91 mg; Calcium: 109.2 mg; Iron: 4.6 mg; Vit. D: 0 mcg; Vit. B$_{12}$: 0 mcg

---

Easy Vegan French Toast

Instead of drowning your French toast in powdered sugar and maple syrup, use a healthier sugar-free jam or some agave nectar for a healthier, yet still sweet topping. **Serves 4**

35/106 each

2 bananas	1 t. cinnamon
½ c. soy milk	½ t. nutmeg
1 T. orange juice	Oil or vegan margarine for frying
1 T. maple syrup	
¾ t. vanilla	12 thick slices bread
1 T. flour	

1. Using a blender or mixer, mix together the bananas, soy milk, orange juice, maple syrup, and vanilla until smooth and creamy.
2. Whisk in flour, cinnamon, and nutmeg, and pour into a pie plate or shallow pan.
3. Heat 1–2 T. of vegan margarine or oil in a large skillet.

Bell Peppers Stuffed with Couscous

Baked stuffed peppers are always a hit with those who appreciate presentation, and this recipe takes very little effort. **Serves 4**

4 c. water or vegetable broth	2 green onions, sliced
3 c. couscous	½ t. cumin
2 T. olive oil	½ t. chili powder
2 T. lemon or lime juice	4 green bell peppers
1 c. frozen peas or corn, thawed	

1. Preheat oven to 350°F.
2. Bring water or vegetable broth to a boil and add couscous. Cover, turn off heat, and let sit for 10–15 minutes, until couscous is cooked. Fluff with a fork.
3. Combine couscous with olive oil, lemon or lime juice, peas or corn, green onions, cumin, and chili powder.
4. Cut the tops off the bell peppers, and remove seeds.
5. Stuff couscous into bell peppers and place the tops back on, using a toothpick to secure, if needed.
6. Transfer to a baking dish and bake for 15 minutes.

Sunday

Glasses of Water Consumed: _____

Thoughts About Today: _____

_____

_____

What I Ate Today

Time	Food Item	Amount	Calories	Fat	Carbs	Fiber	Protein
TOTAL							

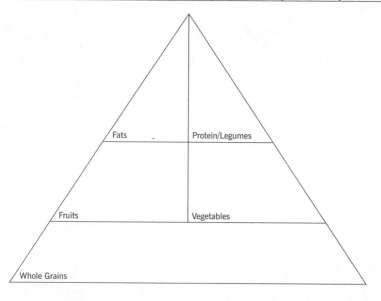

WEEK 1 IN REVIEW

I feel: _____

_____

_____

_____

My greatest food discovery this week was: _____

_____

_____

_____

This week's biggest vegan challenge was: _____

_____

_____

_____

New food I'd like to try: _____

_____

_____

_____

When I look back at this week, I most want to remember: _____

_____

_____

_____

Nutrition Totals

	Calories	Fat	Carbs	Fiber	Protein
Goal					
Actual					

WEEK 2

You made it through Week 1! How are you feeling? You should feel proud of yourself. Now that you know you can do it, Week 2 is going to be even easier. This week, we'll try out some new foods (just a few), such as tofu and dairy substitutes, and you may start to notice some changes in your body. If you're used to eating a diet heavy in meats, dairy, and processed foods, your body will be adjusting to this new easily digestible and nutritious diet—not to mention all the extra fiber you're getting! This may lead to feelings of bloating, or even feeling grumpy. Think of these as sort of food withdrawal symptoms, because that's exactly what they are. The solution? Drink lots of water, grab a healthy snack, and let the feelings pass. Have a favorite movie handy to distract you, or catch up with a friend over tea.

On the other hand, now is the time when you might begin feeling absolutely divine! Most people find that during the first couple of weeks of eating vegan they feel "lighter" or less sluggish mentally and physically. Food is moving through your digestive system more quickly, your body is happy with the abundance of nourishment it's receiving, and all those extra nutrients are flooding your system with energy. Is your skin a little brighter? Nails a little stronger? Are your pants a little looser? If not yet, they just may be by the end of this week!

Monday

Breakfast

1 (3-inch) bagel with 2 T. hummus, 1 small banana, 1 c. tomato juice (no salt added)

Cal.: 326.9; Fat: 4.1 g; Protein: 11 g; Sodium: 393.3 mg; Fiber: 6.7 g; Carbs.: 66.6 g; Sugar: 23.9 g; Zinc: 2.3 mg; Calcium: 91.5 mg; Iron: 5.5 mg; Vit. D: 0 mcg; Vit. B_{12}: 0 mcg

Lunch

1¾ c. Greek Salad with Tofu with 1 c. romaine lettuce

Cal.: 347.; Fat: 26.1 g; Protein: 16.6 g; Sodium: 509 mg; Fiber: 5.6 g; Carbs.: 19.5 g; Sugar: 8.3 g; Zinc: 1.7 mg; Calcium: 608.5 mg; Iron: 3.5 mg; Vit. D: 0 mcg; Vit. B_{12}: 0 mcg

Snack

1 small apple, 1 oz. almonds

Cal.: 238.5; Fat: 14.1 g; Protein: 6.3 g; Sodium: 1.8 mg; Fiber: 7 g; Carbs.: 26.7 g; Sugar: 16.6 g; Zinc: 1 mg; Calcium: 82.8 mg; Iron: 1.2 mg; Vit. D: 0 mcg; Vit. B_{12}: 0 mcg

Dinner

1 oz. Sun-Dried Tomato Pesto with 1 c. whole grain pasta, 1 c. steamed spinach with 16 g nutritional yeast

Cal.: 358.4; Fat: 9.8 g; Protein: 24.8 g; Sodium: 387.2 mg; Fiber: 15.6 g; Carbs.: 51.98 g; Sugar: 3.9 g; Zinc: 5.5 mg; Calcium: 289 mg; Iron: 9.6 mg; Vit. D: 0 mcg; Vit. B_{12}: 7.8 mcg

Greek Salad with Tofu

Serves 3

¼ c. olive oil
2 T. balsamic vinegar
1 t. basil
½ t. oregano
½ t. salt
½ t. black pepper
1 block firm tofu, well-pressed and cut into 1-inch cubes

2 tomatoes, sliced
1 red or yellow bell pepper, chopped
1 large or 2 small cucumbers, sliced
½ red onion, diced
¼ c. Kalamata olives

1. Whisk together the olive oil, vinegar, basil, oregano, and salt and pepper. Add cut tofu, covering well with dressing. Allow it to marinate for at least 1 hour.
2. Add remaining ingredients and gently toss to combine well.

Sun-Dried Tomato Pesto

Yields 1 cup

⅓ c. sun-dried tomatoes
2 c. fresh basil leaves
½ c. pine nuts or walnuts
3 cloves garlic

¼ c. nutritional yeast
½ t. salt
¼ t. black pepper
¼ c. olive oil

1. If using dehydrated sun-dried tomatoes, reconstitute in water until soft and pliable, about 15 minutes.
2. Puree together all ingredients, adding oil last to achieve desired consistency.

Glasses of Water Consumed: _____

Thoughts About Today: _____

_____

_____

What I Ate Today

Time	Food Item	Amount	Calories	Fat	Carbs	Fiber	Protein
TOTAL							

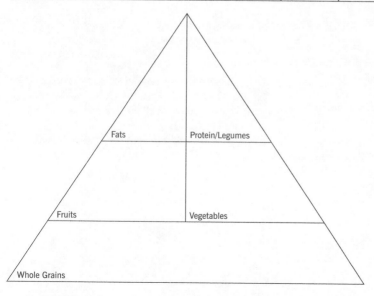

Tuesday

Breakfast

2 c. Strawberry Protein Smoothie, 1 c. chocolate soy milk

Cal.: 324; Fat: 8 g; Protein: 15 g; Sodium: 153 mg; Fiber: 6.3 g; Carbs.: 53 g; Sugar: 36 g; Zinc: 1.98 mg; Calcium: 462 mg; Iron: 2.88 mg; Vit. D: 0 mcg; Vit. B$_{12}$: 3 mcg

Lunch

Vegetarian sandwich with 1 oz. Sun-Dried Tomato Pesto (see recipe in Week 2, Mon.), 1 oz. avocado, tomato slices, and sprouts on whole grain bread, 1 c. tomato juice (no salt added), 3 oz. baby carrots with 1 T. hummus

Cal.: 523.33; Fat: 16.95 g; Protein: 20.38 g; Sodium: 691.65 mg; Fiber: 13.58 g; Carbs.: 80.6 g; Sugar: 44 g; Zinc: 1.85 mg; Calcium: 489.88 mg; Iron: 4.88 mg; Vit. D: 0 mcg; Vit. B$_{12}$: 0.41 mcg

Snack

200 calories of whole grain chips with ¼ c. Black Bean Guacamole

Record nutritional values for your choice of whole grain chips in today's journal. The following nutritional values are for the Black Bean Guacamole alone.

Cal.: 118; Fat: 3.9 g; Protein: 5.6 g; Sodium: 34 mg; Fiber: 5.2 g; Carbs.: 17 g; Sugar: 1 g; Zinc: 1.2 mg; Calcium: 33 mg; Iron: 1.4 mg; Vit. D: 0 mcg; Vit. B$_{12}$: 0 mcg

Dinner

1½ c. Curried Rice and Lentils

Cal.: 543; Fat: 3 g; Protein: 22.5 g; Sodium: 16.5 mg; Fiber: 25.5 g; Carbs.: 37.5 g; Sugar: 6 g; Zinc: 3 mg; Calcium: 76.5 mg; Iron: 7.5 mg; Vit. D: 0 mcg; Vit. B$_{12}$: 0 mcg

Strawberry Protein Smoothie

Serves 2

½ c. frozen strawberries
½ block silken tofu
1 banana

¾ c. orange juice
3–4 ice cubes
1 T. agave nectar (optional)

Blend together all ingredients until smooth and creamy.

Black Bean Guacamole

Yields 2 cups

1 (15-oz.) can black beans
3 avocados
1 T. lime juice
3 scallions, chopped
1 large tomato, diced

2 cloves garlic, minced
½ t. chili powder
¼ t. salt
1 T. chopped fresh cilantro

1. Using a fork or a potato masher, mash the beans in a medium-sized bowl just until they are halfway mashed, leaving some texture.
2. Combine all the remaining ingredients, and mash together until mixed.
3. Adjust seasonings to taste.

4. Allow to sit for at least 10 minutes before serving to allow the flavors to set.
5. Gently mix again just before serving.

Curried Rice and Lentils

Serves 4

1½ c. white or brown rice
1 c. lentils
2 tomatoes, diced
3½ c. water or vegetable broth

1 T. curry powder
½ t. cumin
½ t. turmeric
½ t. garlic powder
Salt and pepper, to taste

1. Combine all ingredients except salt and pepper in a large soup or stockpot. Bring to a slow simmer, then cover and cook for 20 minutes, stirring occasionally, until rice is done and liquid is absorbed.
2. Taste, then add a bit of salt and pepper if needed.

Tuesday

Glasses of Water Consumed: _____

Thoughts About Today: _____

_____

_____

What I Ate Today

Time	Food Item	Amount	Calories	Fat	Carbs	Fiber	Protein
TOTAL							

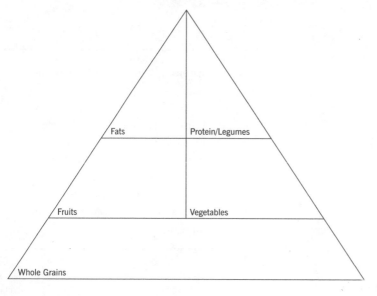

Fats

Protein/Legumes

Fruits

Vegetables

Whole Grains

Wednesday

Breakfast

¾ c. whole grain cereal, 1 c. soy milk, 1 c. sliced fresh pineapple

Cal.: 260.83; Fat: 3.12 g; Protein: 7.07 g; Sodium: 269.53 mg; Fiber: 6.9 g; Carbs.: 55.03 g; Sugar: 23.47 g; Zinc: 20.2 mg; Calcium: 1394.83 mg; Iron: 25.2 mg; Vit. D: 54.7 mcg; Vit. B$_{12}$: 8.18 mcg

Lunch

1½ c. leftover Curried Rice and Lentils (see recipe in Week 2, Tues.) with 1 medium tomato added

Cal.: 565.1; Fat: 3.2 g; Protein: 23.6 g; Sodium: 22.7 mg; Fiber: 27 g; Carbs.: 72.3 g; Sugar: 9.2 g; Zinc: 3.2 mg; Calcium: 88.8 mg; Iron: 7.8 mg; Vit. D: 0 mcg; Vit. B$_{12}$: 0 mcg .

Snack

½ bagel with 1 T. hummus

Cal.: 98; Fat: 1.85 g; Protein: 4.05 g; Sodium: 184.3 mg; Fiber: 1.55 g; Carbs.: 16.6 g; Sugar: 1.45 g; Zinc: 0.85 mg; Calcium: 31.05 mg; Iron: 2.1 mg; Vit. D: 0 mcg; Vit. B$_{12}$: 0 mcg

Dinner

½ block Easy Barbecue Baked Tofu, 1 medium steamed sweet potato, side green salad with 2 c. romaine lettuce, 1 tomato, and 1 diced cucumber, 2 T. Goddess Dressing (see recipe in Week 1, Mon.)

Cal.: 679.2; Fat: 27.2 g; Protein: 1154.2 g; Sodium: 11.32 mg; Fiber: 86.3 g; Carbs.: 86.3 g; Sugar: 47.66 g; Zinc: 4.98 mg; Calcium: 1268.3 mg; Iron: 8.52 mg; Vit. D: 0 mcg; Vit. B$_{12}$: 0 mcg

Easy Barbecue Baked Tofu

Serves 2

1 container firm or extra-firm tofu, well pressed

Barbecue sauce, any kind, about ¾ c.

1. Preheat oven to 350°F. Slice tofu into squares or strips about ¾ inch thick.
2. Brush a layer of barbecue sauce on a baking tray or cookie sheet. Arrange tofu slices in a single layer, and brush well with a generous layer of barbecue sauce.
3. Bake for 30–40 minutes or until tofu is lightly crisped and sauce is baked on. Serve topped with extra sauce, if preferred.

Shaken, Not Stirred Before you pour that glass of orange juice (or soy milk), shake it up! The calcium in these drinks tends to settle at the bottom of the carton, so to get the best bone-boosting effect, shake before you drink. If you're a heavy smoker or coffee drinker, consider taking a supplement, as these inhibit absorption of several nutrients.

Glasses of Water Consumed: _____

Thoughts About Today: _____

_____

_____

What I Ate Today

Time	Food Item	Amount	Calories	Fat	Carbs	Fiber	Protein
TOTAL							

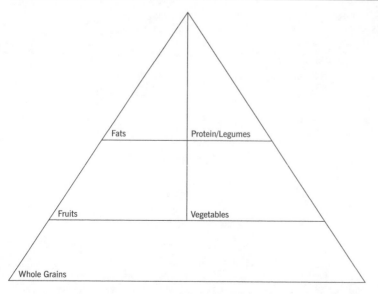

Fats

Protein/Legumes

Fruits

Vegetables

Whole Grains

Thursday

Breakfast

Tortilla wrap with 1 T. nondairy cream cheese and sliced strawberries, 1 c. chocolate soy milk

Cal.: 329; Fat: 12.1 g; Protein: 13.4 g; Sodium: 337 mg; Fiber: 6 g; Carbs.: 43.5 g; Sugar: 8.9 g; Zinc: 0.2 mg; Calcium: 211.7 mg; Iron: 3.18 mg; Vit. D: 3 mcg; Vit. B$_{12}$: 0.36 mcg

Lunch

Barbecue tofu sandwiches from leftover Easy Barbecue Baked Tofu (see recipe in Week 2, Wed.) with 1 T. vegan mayonnaise, ¼ tomato, sliced, and ¼ c. iceberg lettuce, 1 small apple, 1 c. soy milk

Cal.: 413.15; Fat: 16.58 g; Protein: 24.93 g; Sodium: 671.35 mg; Fiber: 6.1 g; Carbs.: 44.08 g; Sugar: 1 g; Zinc: 2.08 mg; Calcium: 663.93 mg; Iron: 4.65 mg; Vit. D: 3 mcg; Vit. B$_{12}$: 0.36 mcg

Snack

1 c. popcorn with 16 g nutritional yeast

Cal.: 75.6; Fat: 0.8 g; Protein: 9 g; Sodium: 5.3 mg; Fiber: 5.2 g; Carbs.: 11.2 g; Sugar: 1.0 g; Zinc: 3.3 mg; Calcium: 0.8 mg; Iron: 0.9 mg; Vit. D: 0 mcg; Vit. B$_{12}$: 7.8 mcg

Dinner

2 Portabella and Pepper Fajitas topped with ½ c. vegetable salsa and 2 T. vegan sour cream, 1 c. steamed broccoli

Cal.: 546; Fat: 21.36 g; Protein: 17.3 g; Sodium: 711 mg; Fiber: 12.6 g; Carbs.: 74.6 g; Sugar: 14.9 g; Zinc: 1.46 mg; Calcium: 190 mg; Iron: 5.6 mg; Vit. D: 0 mcg; Vit. B$_{12}$: 0 mcg

Portabella and Pepper Fajitas

Serves 2

2 T. olive oil

2 large portabella mushrooms, cut into strips

1 green bell pepper, cut into strips

1 red bell pepper, cut into strips

1 onion, cut into strips

¾ t. chili powder

¼ t. cumin

Dash hot sauce (optional)

1 T. chopped fresh cilantro (optional)

4 flour tortillas, warmed

Toppings: vegan sour cream, salsa, avocado, etc.

1. Heat olive oil in a large skillet and add mushrooms, bell peppers, and onion. Allow to cook for 3–5 minutes, until vegetables are almost done.
2. Add chili powder, cumin, and hot sauce, and stir to combine. Cook for 2–3 more minutes, until mushrooms and peppers are soft. Remove from heat and stir in fresh cilantro.
3. Layer the mushrooms and peppers in flour tortillas, and top with nondairy sour cream, salsa, or fresh sliced avocados.

Glasses of Water Consumed: _____

Thoughts About Today: _____

_____

_____

What I Ate Today

Time	Food Item	Amount	Calories	Fat	Carbs	Fiber	Protein
TOTAL							

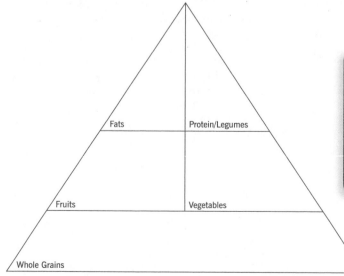

Cooking for Omnivores? If your family still insists on eating a bit of meat, no need to cook two separate meals. Prepare a portion of meat separately, and add it into only a portion of an otherwise vegan soup, pasta, or casserole.

Friday

Breakfast

1½ c. Tropical Breakfast Couscous, 1 banana

Cal.: 526.9; Fat: 25.3 g; Protein: 8.1 g; Sodium: 22 mg; Fiber: 3.6 g; Carbs.: 74.1 g; Sugar: 34.4 g; Zinc: 2.2 mg; Calcium: 43.1 mg; Iron: 1.7 mg; Vit. D: 0 mcg; Vit. B$_{12}$: 0 mcg

Snack

1 slice whole grain toast with ½ T. peanut butter

Cal.: 119.1; Fat: 5.1 g; Protein: 6 g; Sodium: 111.5 mg; Fiber: 2.4 g; Carbs.: 12.8 g; Sugar: 2.2 g; Zinc: 0.4 mg; Calcium: 26.6 mg; Iron: 0.7 mg; Vit. D: 0 mcg; Vit. B$_{12}$: 0 mcg

Lunch

1⅛ c. Spicy Southwestern Two Bean Salad, 1 small apple, 1 c. orange juice

Cal.: 479.5; Fat: 17.3 g; Protein: 10.9 g; Sodium: 620.5 mg; Fiber: 13.2 g; Carbs.: 77.6 g; Sugar: 38.7 g; Zinc: 1.7 mg; Calcium: 427.9 mg; Iron: 4.45 mg; Vit. D: 0 mcg; Vit. B$_{12}$: 0.41 mcg

Dinner

1 c. Artichoke and Olive Puttanesca, 1 c. steamed spinach

Cal.: 495.4; Fat: 14.5 g; Protein: 18.3 g; Sodium: 790 mg; Fiber: 9.9 g; Carbs.: 81.7 g; Sugar: 2.5 g; Zinc: 1.4 mg; Calcium: 292 mg; Iron: 10.6 mg; Vit. D: 0 mcg; Vit. B$_{12}$: 0 mcg

Tropical Breakfast Couscous

Serves 2

1 c. coconut milk
1 c. pineapple juice or orange juice
1 c. couscous
½ t. vanilla
2 T. maple syrup or agave nectar
Sliced fresh fruit (optional)

1. In a small saucepan, heat coconut milk and juice until just about to simmer. Do not boil.
2. Add couscous and heat for one minute. Stir in vanilla, cover, and turn off heat. Allow to sit, covered, for 5 minutes, until couscous is cooked.
3. Fluff couscous with a fork and stir in maple syrup. Garnish with fresh fruit.

Spicy Southwestern Two Bean Salad

Serves 6

1 (15-oz.) can black beans, drained and rinsed
1 (15-oz.) can kidney beans, drained and rinsed
1 red or yellow bell pepper, chopped
1 large tomato, diced
⅔ c. corn (fresh, canned, or frozen)
1 red onion, diced
⅓ c. olive oil
¼ c. lime juice
½ t. chili powder
½ t. garlic powder
¼ t. cayenne pepper
½ t. salt
¼ c. chopped fresh cilantro

1. In a large bowl, combine the black beans, kidney beans, bell pepper, tomato, corn, and onion.
2. In a separate small bowl, whisk together the olive oil, lime juice, chili powder, garlic powder, cayenne pepper, and salt.
3. Pour over bean mixture, tossing to coat. Stir in fresh cilantro.
4. Chill for at least 1 hour before serving, to allow flavors to mingle. Gently toss again just before serving.

Artichoke and Olive Puttanesca

Serves 4

3 cloves garlic, minced
2 T. olive oil
1 (14-oz.) can diced or crushed tomatoes
¼ c. sliced black olives
¼ c. sliced green olives
1 c. chopped artichoke hearts
2 T. capers
½ t. red pepper flakes
½ t. basil
¾ t. parsley
¼ t. salt
1 (12-oz.) package pasta, prepared

1. Heat garlic in olive oil for 2–3 minutes. Reduce heat and add remaining ingredients, except pasta.
2. Cook over low heat, uncovered, for 10–12 minutes, until most of the liquid from tomatoes is absorbed.
3. Toss with cooked pasta.

Friday

Glasses of Water Consumed: _____

Thoughts About Today: _____

_____

_____

What I Ate Today

Time	Food Item	Amount	Calories	Fat	Carbs	Fiber	Protein
TOTAL							

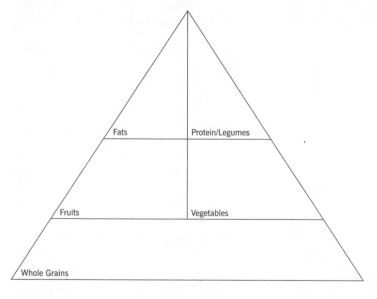

Fats

Protein/Legumes

Fruits

Vegetables

Whole Grains

Saturday

Breakfast

1 c. Chili Masala Tofu Scramble

Cal.: 313.5; Fat: 21 g; Protein: 21.75 g; Sodium: 395.25 mg; Fiber: 4.05 g; Carbs.: 12 g; Sugar: 1.5 g; Zinc: 2.7 mg; Calcium: 843.75 mg; Iron: 4.88 mg; Vit. D: 0 mcg; Vit. B_{12}: 0 mcg

Lunch

1 c. leftover Artichoke and Olive Puttanesca (see recipe in Week 2, Fri.)

Cal.: 454; Fat: 14 g; Protein: 13 g; Sodium: 790 mg; Fiber: 5.6 g; Carbs.: 75 g; Sugar: 1.7 g; Zinc: 0 mg; Calcium: 47 mg; Iron: 4.2 mg; Vit. D: 0 mcg; Vit. B_{12}: 0 mcg

Snack

1 medium apple, sliced, with ½ T. peanut butter and ½ oz. raisins

Cal.: 169.35; Fat: 4.35 g; Protein: 3.35 g; Sodium: 4.55 mg; Fiber: 4.6 g; Carbs.: 33.2 g; Sugar: 24.3 g; Zinc: 0.15 mg; Calcium: 15.9 mg; Iron: 0.45 mg; Vit. D: 0 mcg; Vit. B_{12}: 0 mcg

Dinner

7 oz. Cuban Black Beans, Sweet Potatoes, and Rice, 1 c. steamed broccoli

Cal.: 584; Fat: 7 g; Protein: 32.3 g; Sodium: 33 mg; Fiber: 24.6 g; Carbs.: 103.1 g; Sugar: 6.3 g; Zinc: 5.5 mg; Calcium: 226 mg; Iron: 7.8 mg; Vit. D: 0 mcg; Vit. B_{12}: 0.1 mcg

Chili Masala Tofu Scramble

Tofu scramble is an easy and versatile vegan breakfast. This version adds chili and curry for subcontinental flavor. Toss in whatever veggies you have on hand—tomatoes, spinach, or diced broccoli would work well. **Serves 2**

1 block firm or extra-firm tofu, pressed	¾ c. sliced mushrooms
1 small onion, diced	1 T. soy sauce
2 cloves garlic, minced	1 t. curry powder
2 T. olive oil	½ t. cumin
1 small red chili pepper, minced	¼ t. turmeric
1 green bell pepper, chopped	1 t. nutritional yeast (optional)

1. Cut or crumble pressed tofu into 1-inch cubes.
2. Sauté onion and garlic in olive oil for a minute or two, until onion is soft.
3. Add tofu, chili pepper, bell pepper, and mushrooms, stirring well to combine.
4. Add remaining ingredients, except nutritional yeast, and combine well. Allow to cook until tofu is lightly browned, about 6–8 minutes.
5. Remove from heat and stir in nutritional yeast if desired.

Cuban Black Beans, Sweet Potatoes, and Rice

Stir some plain steamed rice right into the pot, or serve it alongside these well-seasoned beans. **Serves 6**

3 cloves garlic, minced	1 T. chili powder
2 large sweet potatoes, chopped small	1 t. paprika
	1 t. cumin
2 T. olive oil	1 T. lime juice
2 (15-oz.) cans black beans, drained	Hot sauce, to taste
¾ c. vegetable broth	2 c. cooked rice

1. In a large skillet or soup pot, sauté garlic and sweet potatoes in olive oil for 2–3 minutes.
2. Reduce heat to medium low and add beans, vegetable broth, chili powder, paprika, and cumin. Bring to a simmer, cover, and allow to cook for 25–30 minutes, until sweet potatoes are soft.
3. Stir in lime juice and hot sauce, to taste. Serve hot over rice.

Glasses of Water Consumed: _____

Thoughts About Today: _____

_____

_____

What I Ate Today

Time	Food Item	Amount	Calories	Fat	Carbs	Fiber	Protein
TOTAL							

Fats

Protein/Legumes

Fruits

Vegetables

Whole Grains

Wrap It Up Leftover tofu scramble makes an excellent lunch, or wrap leftovers (or planned-overs!) in a warmed flour tortilla to make breakfast-style burritos, perhaps with some salsa or beans. Why isn't it called "scrambled tofu" instead of "tofu scramble" if it's a substitute for scrambled eggs? This is one of the great conundrums of veganism.

Breakfast

2 oz. store-bought polenta pan-fried in 1 t. oil, with ½ c. salsa, 1 c. orange juice

Cal.: 312; Fat: 2 g; Protein: 6.6 g; Sodium: 19.6 mg; Fiber: 4 g; Carbs.: 69 g; Sugar: 22.4 g; Zinc: 1 mg; Calcium: 353.4 mg; Iron: 4.25 mg; Vit. D: 0 mcg; Vit. B$_{12}$: 0.41 mcg

Lunch

7 oz. leftover Cuban Black Beans, Sweet Potatoes, and Rice (see recipe in Week 2, Sat.)

Cal.: 535; Fat: 6.4 g; Protein: 29 g; Sodium: 33 mg; Fiber: 20 g; Carbs.: 93 g; Sugar: 4.4 g; Zinc: 4.9 mg; Calcium: 170 mg; Iron: 6.9 mg; Vit. D: 0 mcg; Vit. B$_{12}$: 0.1 mcg

Snack

175 calories of whole grain chips with ¼ c. leftover Black Bean Guacamole (see recipe in Week 2, Tues.)

Record nutritional values for your choice of whole grain chips in today's journal. The following nutritional values are for the Black Bean Guacamole (see recipe in Week 2, Tuesday) alone.

Cal.: 118; Fat: 3.9 g; Protein: 5.6 g; Sodium: 34 mg; Fiber: 5.2 g; Carbs.: 17 g; Sugar: 1 g; Zinc: 1.2 mg; Calcium: 33 mg; Iron: 1.4 mg; Vit. D: 0 mcg; Vit. B$_{12}$: 0 mcg

Dinner

1½ c. Basic Tofu Lasagna, side green salad with 2 c. romaine lettuce, 1 tomato, and 1 diced cucumber, 2 T. Goddess Dressing (see recipe in Week 1, Mon.)

Cal.: 662.2; Fat: 20.3 g; Protein: 33.5 g; Sodium: 2151.2 mg; Fiber: 10.32 g; Carbs.: 95.9 g; Sugar: 18.26 g; Zinc: 3.18 mg; Calcium: 577.5 mg; Iron: 10.12 mg; Vit. D: 0 mcg; Vit. B$_{12}$: 0.12 mcg

Basic Tofu Lasagna

Seasoned tofu takes the place of ricotta cheese, and it really does look and taste like the real thing. Fresh parsley adds flavor, and with store-bought sauce, it's quick to get in the oven. **Serves 6**

1 block firm tofu	2 t. basil
1 (12-oz.) block silken tofu	3 T. chopped fresh parsley
¼ c. nutritional yeast	1 t. salt
1 T. lemon juice	1 (16-oz.) package lasagna noodles
1 T. soy sauce	4 c. spaghetti sauce
1 t. garlic powder	

1. In a large bowl, mash together the firm tofu, silk tofu, nutritional yeast, lemon juice, soy sauce, garlic, basil, parsley, and salt until combined and crumbly like ricotta cheese.
2. Preheat oven to 350°F.
3. To assemble the lasagna, spread about ⅔ cup tomato sauce on the bottom of a lasagna pan, then add a layer of noodles.
4. Spread about half of the tofu mixture on top of the noodles, followed by another layer of sauce. Place a second layer of noodles on top, followed by the remaining tofu and more sauce. Finish it off with a third layer of noodles and the rest of the sauce.
5. Cover and bake for 25 minutes.

Date ____ / ____ / ____

Glasses of Water Consumed: _____

Thoughts About Today: _____

_____

_____

What I Ate Today

Time	Food Item	Amount	Calories	Fat	Carbs	Fiber	Protein
TOTAL							

Fats
Protein/Legumes
Fruits
Vegetables
Whole Grains

Ready-to-Go Polenta Look for prepared polenta in a tube at the grocery store. This store-bought polenta is already cooked, so all you need to do is fry it up in a sauté pan with a bit of oil. For extra protein, add a few spoonfuls of black beans to the salsa.

WEEK 2 IN REVIEW

I feel: _____

_____

_____

_____

My greatest food discovery this week was: _____

_____

_____

_____

This week's biggest vegan challenge was: _____

_____

_____

_____

New food I'd like to try: _____

_____

_____

_____

When I look back at this week, I most want to remember: _____

_____

_____

_____

Nutrition Totals

	Calories	Fat	Carbs	Fiber	Protein
Goal					
Actual					

WEEK 3

By now, you've gotten used to cooking at home a bit more, and the excitement and newness of it all may have started to wear off as you begin settling into your new routine. Focus on small, positive changes to keep you motivated this week. Browse through your notes from Week 1 and look at just how far you've come! You've already been vegan for two whole weeks now! Wasn't it easy?

Eating vegan will begin to seem more normal to you now, and your friends and family will soon stop paying attention to your new habits. But don't let this new daily grind get you down—you've still got lots of new food options to explore. You've tried tofu a few times, and you know what great variety the vegetable kingdom has to offer. Now you're ready to expand your options even further. This week, we'll continue experimenting with tofu, and try a few other new foods, too. Are you ready to try some mock meats?

Give your taste buds a chance to adjust to the newness of meat substitutes. Some are startlingly similar to the real deal in flavor and texture, while others are quite tasty, but won't fool anyone. Not all mock meats are the same, so try a few different brands to find one that you like, or vary your preparation technique. For example, if you find you don't like microwaved vegan sausage patties, try pan-frying them in a bit of oil.

Monday

Breakfast

1 English muffin with 1 vegetarian sausage patty, ¼ medium tomato, and 2 (1-oz.) avocado slices, 1 c. soy milk

Cal.: 421.98; Fat: 16.85 g; Protein: 26.88 g; Sodium: 542.55 mg; Fiber: 8.88 g; Carbs.: 41.4 g; Sugar: 5 g; Zinc: 1.15 mg; Calcium: 194.88 mg; Iron: 5.72 mg; Vit. D: 3 mcg; Vit. B_{12}: 2.46 mcg

Lunch

1 baked potato with 2 T. vegan sour cream and ½ c. frozen mixed veggies

Record nutritional values for your choice of frozen mixed veggies in today's journal. The nutritional values below are for the baked potato and vegan sour cream only.
Cal.: 165; Fat: 21 g; Protein: 6.5 g; Sodium: 85 mg; Fiber: 3 g; Carbs.: 30.2 g; Sugar: 1.6 g; Zinc: 0.5 mg; Calcium: 20.7 mg; Iron: 1.5 mg; Vit. D: 0 mcg; Vit. B_{12}: 0 mcg

Snack

2 oz. almonds, 1 oz. dried apricots, 1 c. orange juice

Cal.: 499.5; Fat: 27.7 g; Protein: 14.7 g; Sodium: 3.4 mg; Fiber: 8.8 g; Carbs.: 55.7 g; Sugar: 39.2 g; Zinc: 1.9 mg; Calcium: 513.2 mg; Iron: 2.7 mg; Vit. D: 0 mcg; Vit. B_{12}: 0.41 mcg

Dinner

1½ c. Potatoes "Au Gratin" Casserole, 1 c. Maple-Glazed Roast Veggies

Cal.: 574; Fat: 10.5 g; Protein: 14.4 g; Sodium: 764 mg; Fiber: 13.1 g; Carbs.: 105 g; Sugar: 23 g; Zinc: 2.04 mg; Calcium: 298 mg; Iron: 6 mg; Vit. D: 0 mcg; Vit. B_{12}: 1.6 mcg

Potatoes "Au Gratin" Casserole

Serves 4

4 potatoes	1 t. garlic powder
1 onion, chopped	2 T. nutritional yeast
1 T. vegan margarine	1 t. lemon juice
2 T. flour	½ t. salt
2 c. unsweetened soy milk	¾ t. paprika
2 t. onion powder	½ t. pepper

1. Preheat oven to 375°F.
2. Slice potatoes into thin coins and arrange half the slices in a casserole or baking dish. Layer half of the onion on top of the potatoes.
3. Melt the margarine over low heat and add flour, stirring to make a paste. Add soy milk, onion powder, garlic powder, nutritional yeast, lemon juice, and salt, stirring to combine. Stir over low heat until sauce has thickened, about 2–3 minutes.
4. Pour half of sauce over potatoes and onions, then layer the remaining potatoes and onions on top of the sauce. Pour the remaining sauce on top.
5. Sprinkle with paprika and pepper.
6. Cover and bake for 45 minutes, and an additional 10 minutes, uncovered.

Maple-Glazed Roast Veggies

Serves 5

3 carrots, chopped	⅓ c. maple syrup
2 small parsnips, chopped	2 T. Dijon mustard
2 sweet potatoes, chopped	1 T. balsamic vinegar
2 T. olive oil	½ t. hot sauce
Salt and pepper to taste	

1. Preheat oven to 400°F.
2. On a large baking sheet, spread out chopped carrots, parsnips, and sweet potatoes. Drizzle with olive oil and season generously with salt and pepper. Roast for 40 minutes, tossing once.
3. In a small bowl, whisk together maple syrup, Dijon mustard, balsamic vinegar, hot sauce, and salt and pepper.
4. Transfer the roasted vegetables to a large bowl and toss well with the maple mixture.

Date ____ / ____ / ____

Glasses of Water Consumed: _____

Thoughts About Today: _____

_____

_____

What I Ate Today

Time	Food Item	Amount	Calories	Fat	Carbs	Fiber	Protein
TOTAL							

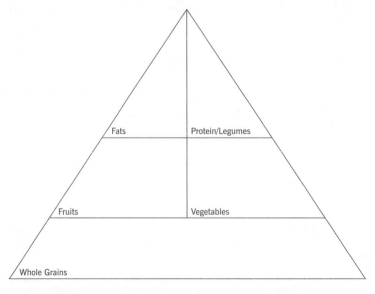

Fats

Protein/Legumes

Fruits

Vegetables

Whole Grains

Tuesday

Breakfast

¾ c. whole grain cereal, 1 c. soy milk, 1 small banana

Cal.: 268.23; Fat: 3.22 g; Protein: 7.27 g; Sodium: 268.83 mg; Fiber: 7.2 g; Carbs.: 56.53 g; Sugar: 19.57 g; Zinc: 20.2 mg; Calcium: 1378.43 mg; Iron: 25 mg; Vit. D: 54.7 mcg; Vit. B$_{12}$: 8.18 mcg

Lunch

1 c. leftover Maple-Glazed Roast Veggies (see recipe in Week 3, Mon.), store-bought tomato soup (about 250 calories)

Record nutritional values for your choice of tomato soup in today's journal. The nutritional values below are for the Maple-Glazed Roast Veggies only.

Cal.: 233; Fat: 5.5 g; Protein: 2.4 g; Sodium: 91 mg; Fiber: 7.4 g; Carbs.: 44 g; Sugar: 22 g; Zinc: 1.5 mg; Calcium: 79 mg; Iron: 1.5 mg; Vit. D: 0 mcg; Vit. B$_{12}$: 0 mcg

Snack

1 oz. banana chips

Cal.: 145; Fat: 9.4 g; Protein: 0.6 g; Sodium: 1.7 mg; Fiber: 2.2 g; Carbs.: 16.3 g; Sugar: 9.9 g; Zinc: 0.2 mg; Calcium: 5 mg; Iron: 0.4 mg; Vit. D: 0 mcg; Vit. B$_{12}$: 0 mcg

Dinner

1 Tofu and Portabella Enchilada, ½ c. black beans, side green salad with 2 c. romaine lettuce, 1 tomato, and 1 diced cucumber, 2 T. Goddess Dressing (see recipe in Week 1, Mon.)

Cal.: 565.7; Fat: 24.75 g; Protein: 25.1 g; Sodium: 594.05 mg; Fiber: 16.62 g; Carbs.: 68.3 g; Sugar: 10.76 g; Zinc: 3.53 mg; Calcium: 499.7 mg; Iron: 8.12 mg; Vit. D: 0 mcg; Vit. B$_{12}$: 0 mcg

Tofu and Portabella Enchiladas

Turn up the heat by adding some fresh minced or canned chilies. If you're already addicted to vegan cheese, add a handful of grated cheese to the filling as well as on top. **Serves 8**

1 block firm tofu, diced small	2 T. oil
5 portabella mushrooms, chopped	2 t. chili powder
	½ c. sliced black olives
1 onion, diced	1 (15-oz.) can enchilada sauce
3 cloves garlic, minced	8–10 flour tortillas

1. Preheat oven to 350°F.
2. In a large skillet, heat the tofu, mushrooms, onion, and garlic in oil until tofu is just lightly sautéed, about 4–5 minutes. Add chili powder and heat for one more minute, stirring to coat well.
3. Remove from heat and add black olives and ⅓ cup enchilada sauce, and combine well.
4. Spread a thin layer of enchilada sauce in the bottom of a baking pan or casserole dish.
5. Place about ¼ cup of the tofu and mushrooms in each flour tortilla and roll, placing snugly in the baking dish. Top with remaining enchilada sauce, coating the tops of each tortilla well.
6. Bake for 25–30 minutes.

Date ____ / ____ / ____

Glasses of Water Consumed: _____

Thoughts About Today: _____

_____

_____

What I Ate Today

Time	Food Item	Amount	Calories	Fat	Carbs	Fiber	Protein
TOTAL							

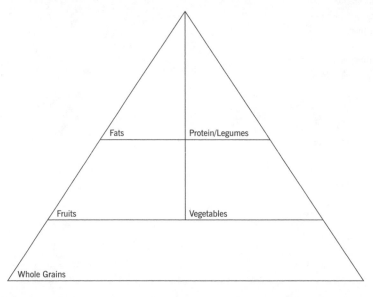

Wednesday

Breakfast

Peanut butter oatmeal (½ c. oatmeal with 1 T. peanut butter), 1 c. chocolate soy milk, 1 small apple

Cal.: 447.5; Fat: 13.8 g; Protein: 15.4 g; Sodium: 144.5 mg; Fiber: 11.6 g; Carbs.: 69.6 g; Sugar: 33.5 g; Zinc: 0.7 mg; Calcium: 308.9 mg; Iron: 2.08 mg; Vit. D: 0 mcg; Vit. B$_{12}$: 3 mcg

Lunch

1 leftover Tofu and Portabella Enchilada (see recipe in Week 3, Tues.), 1 c. tomato juice, 1 banana

Cal.: 379.9; Fat: 12.4 g; Protein: 13.9 g; Sodium: 392.3 mg; Fiber: 6.6 g; Carbs.: 59.4 g; Sugar: 22 g; Zinc: 1.6 mg; Calcium: 362.4 mg; Iron: 4.3 mg; Vit. D: 0 mcg; Vit. B$_{12}$: 0 mcg

Snack

3 oz. baby carrots dipped in 2 T. Goddess Dressing (see recipe in Week 1, Mon.), 1 small banana

Cal.: 149.8; Fat: 11.7 g; Protein: 2.7 g; Sodium: 220 mg; Fiber: 3.62 g; Carbs.: 10.2 g; Sugar: 4.36 g; Zinc: mg; Calcium: mg; Iron: mg; Vit. D: mcg; Vit. B$_{12}$: mcg

Dinner

1 c. Indian Spiced Chickpeas with Spinach, 1 c. brown rice

Cal.: 715; Fat: 14.8 g; Protein: 28 g; Sodium: 258.8 mg; Fiber: 24.5 g; Carbs.: 119.8 g; Sugar: 16.7 g; Zinc: 5.2 mg; Calcium: 177.5 mg; Iron: 9.6 mg; Vit. D: 0 mcg; Vit. B$_{12}$: 0.01 mcg

Indian Spiced Chickpeas with Spinach

This is a mild recipe, suitable for the whole family, but if you want to turn up the heat, toss in some fresh minced chiles or a hearty dash of cayenne pepper. It's enjoyable as is for a side dish, or piled on top of rice or another grain for a main meal. **Serves 3**

1 onion, chopped	3 tomatoes, pureed or ⅔ c. tomato paste
2 cloves garlic, minced	½ t. curry
2 T. vegan margarine	¼ t. turmeric
¾ t. coriander	¼ t. salt
1 t. cumin	1 T. lemon juice
1 (15-oz.) can chickpeas, undrained	1 bunch fresh spinach

1. In a large skillet, sauté onions and garlic in margarine until almost soft, about 2 minutes.
2. Reduce heat to medium low and add coriander and cumin. Toast the spices, stirring, for 1 minute.
3. Add the chickpeas with water, tomatoes, curry, turmeric, and salt, and bring to a slow simmer. Allow to cook until most of the liquid has been absorbed, about 10–12 minutes, stirring occasionally, then add lemon juice.
4. Add spinach and stir to combine. Cook just until spinach begins to wilt, about one minute. Serve immediately.

Wednesday

Glasses of Water Consumed: _____

Thoughts About Today: _____

_____

_____

What I Ate Today

Time	Food Item	Amount	Calories	Fat	Carbs	Fiber	Protein
TOTAL							

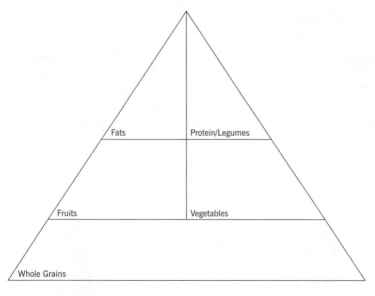

Fats | Protein/Legumes

Fruits | Vegetables

Whole Grains

Thursday

Breakfast

1 c. Pumpkin Protein Smoothie, 1 c. diced pineapple

Cal.: 209.5; Fat: 3 g; Protein: 6.3 g; Sodium: 64.7 mg; Fiber: 4.3 g; Carbs.: 42.6 g; Sugar: 25 g; Zinc: 0.96 mg; Calcium: 266.5 mg; Iron: 2.4 mg; Vit. D: 0 mcg; Vit. B_{12}: 1.5 mcg

Lunch

2 Easy Vegan Pizza Bagels (see recipe in Week 1, Wed.) with 13 slices vegetarian pepperoni

Cal.: 356; Fat: 4 g; Protein: 22 g; Sodium: 778 mg; Fiber: 6 g; Carbs.: 63 g; Sugar: 3 g; Zinc: 1 mg; Calcium: 16 mg; Iron: 4 mg; Vit. D: 0 mcg; Vit. B_{12}: 0 mcg

Snack

2 oz. cashews, 1 c. orange juice

Cal.: 265; Fat: 12.3 g; Protein: 7.1 g; Sodium: 3.4 mg; Fiber: 0.9 g; Carbs.: 35.2 g; Sugar: 23.7 g; Zinc: 1.6 mg; Calcium: 360.4 mg; Iron: 1.9 mg; Vit. D: 0 mcg; Vit. B_{12}: 0.41 mcg

Dinner

1 vegetarian chicken patty burger with ¼ medium tomato, and ¼ c. iceberg lettuce, 1 c. Vegan Ambrosia Fruit Salad, 1 ear corn, 1 c. almond milk

Cal.: 690.25; Fat: 26.68 g; Protein: 23.93 g; Sodium: 1013.35 mg; Fiber: 12.6 g; Carbs.: 101.28 g; Sugar: 23.55 g; Zinc: 2.2 mg; Calcium: 594.93 mg; Iron: 4 mg; Vit. D: 0 mcg; Vit. B_{12}: 0 mcg

Pumpkin Protein Smoothie

Serves 2

½ c. pumpkin puree
1 c. soy milk
¼ c. soy yogurt (plain or vanilla)
1 banana

5–6 ice cubes
¼ t. pumpkin pie spice (or a dash of cinnamon, nutmeg, and allspice)
1 T. maple syrup

Blend all ingredients together until smooth and creamy.

Vegan Ambrosia Fruit Salad

Serves 5

1 (6-oz.) container vegan yogurt, any flavor
1 (20-oz.) can pineapple tidbits, drained
1 apple, chopped small
1 c. grapes, any kind

1 (11-oz.) can mandarin oranges, drained
⅔ c. flaked coconut
½ c. chopped walnuts or pecans (optional)

Gently fold together all ingredients, except nuts. Allow to chill for at least one hour. Carefully stir in nuts just before serving.

Vegan Protein Shakes If you're tempted by those rows of fancy-looking dairy and egg-based protein powders sold at your gym, try a vegan version! Well-stocked natural-foods stores sell a variety of naturally vegan protein powders that you can add to a smoothie for all your muscle-building needs. Look for hemp protein powder or flax meal blends and don't be afraid of the green proteins—some of them are quite tasty!

Glasses of Water Consumed: _____

Thoughts About Today: _____

_____

_____

What I Ate Today

Time	Food Item	Amount	Calories	Fat	Carbs	Fiber	Protein
TOTAL							

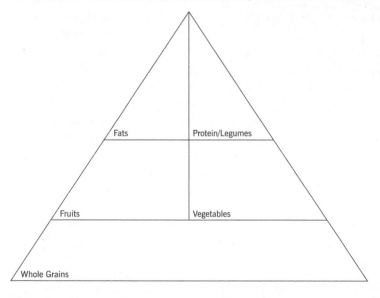

Fats Protein/Legumes

Fruits Vegetables

Whole Grains

Friday

Breakfast

1 c. leftover Vegan Ambrosia Fruit Salad (see recipe in Week 3, Thurs.), soy hot chocolate

Cal.: 309; Fat: 13 g; Protein: 9 g; Sodium: 115 mg; Fiber: 6.2 g; Carbs.: 47 g; Sugar: 33 g; Zinc: 1.14 mg; Calcium: 381 mg; Iron: 1.91 mg; Vit. D: 105 mcg; Vit. B$_{12}$: 2.1 mcg

Lunch

Sandwich with 2 slices vegetarian deli meats, side green salad with 2 c. romaine lettuce, 1 tomato, and 1 diced cucumber, 2 T. Goddess Dressing (see recipe in Week 1, Mon.)

Record nutritional values for your choice of vegetarian deli meats in today's journal. The nutritional values below are for the side green salad and Goddess Dressing only.

Cal.: 203.2; Fat: 12.3 g; Protein: 6.5 g; Sodium: 226.2 mg; Fiber: 6.12 g; Carbs.: 21.9 g; Sugar: 9.76 g; Zinc: 1.58 mg; Calcium: 143.5 mg; Iron: 3.32 mg; Vit. D: 0 mcg; Vit. B$_{12}$: 0 mcg

Snack

Mixed veggies (½ cucumber, 2 oz. baby carrots, ½ c. broccoli) with 2 T. hummus

Cal.: 116.92; Fat: 3.32 g; Protein: 5.38 g; Sodium: 189.5 mg; Fiber: 6.52 g; Carbs.: 19.37 g; Sugar: 6.12 g; Zinc: 1.27 mg; Calcium: 81.63 mg; Iron: 2.18 mg; Vit. D: 0 mcg; Vit. B$_{12}$: 0 mcg

Dinner

¾ c. Baked Teriyaki Tofu Cubes with 1 c. soba noodles

Cal.: 392; Fat: 9.9 g; Protein: 26.8 g; Sodium: 1793.4 mg; Fiber: 2.6 g; Carbs.: 56.4 g; Sugar: 23 g; Zinc: 3.3 mg; Calcium: 763.6 mg; Iron: 4.6 mg; Vit. D: 0 mcg; Vit. B$_{12}$: 0 mcg

Baked Teriyaki Tofu Cubes

Cut tofu into wide slabs or triangular cutlets for a main dish, or smaller cubes to add to a salad, or just for an appetizer or snack. **Serves 3**

⅓ c. soy sauce

3 T. barbecue sauce

2 t. hot chili sauce

¼ c. maple syrup

¾ t. garlic powder

1 block firm or extra-firm tofu, cut into thin chunks

1. Preheat oven to 375°F.
2. In a casserole or baking dish, whisk together the soy sauce, barbecue sauce, chili sauce, maple syrup, and garlic powder.
3. Add tofu, and cover with sauce.
4. Bake for 35–40 minutes, tossing once.

Homemade Baked Tofu It's hard to go wrong with homemade baked tofu. Use just about any store-bought salad dressing, teriyaki sauce, barbecue sauce, or steak marinades. Thicker dressings may need to be thinned with a bit of water first, and to get the best glazing action, make sure there's a bit of sugar added. To save time, you can look for baked tofu in your local grocery store or health-food store—it's ready to go, just heat and eat. Another tip? Most baked tofu recipes will work just as well on an indoor electric grill in about a third of the time.

Friday

Glasses of Water Consumed: _____

Thoughts About Today: _____

_____

_____

What I Ate Today

Time	Food Item	Amount	Calories	Fat	Carbs	Fiber	Protein
TOTAL							

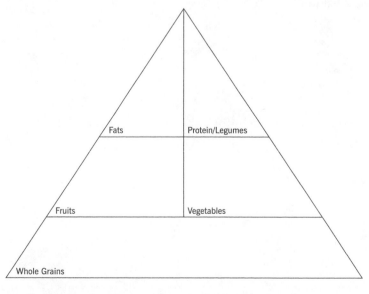

Saturday

Breakfast

1½ c. Chili Masala Tofu Scramble (see recipe in Week 2, Sat.)

Cal.: 418; Fat: 28 g; Protein: 29 g; Sodium: 527 mg; Fiber: 5.4 g; Carbs.: 16 g; Sugar: 2 g; Zinc: 3.6 mg; Calcium: 1125 mg; Iron: 6.5 mg; Vit. D: 0 mcg; Vit. B$_{12}$: 0 mcg

Lunch

1½ c. Sesame Snow Pea Rice Salad

Cal.: 434; Fat: 22 g; Protein: 8 g; Sodium: 1584 mg; Fiber: 2.4 g; Carbs.: 54 g; Sugar: 2.6 g; Zinc: 0 mg; Calcium: 54 mg; Iron: 3 mg; Vit. D: 0 mcg; Vit. B$_{12}$: 0 mcg

Snack

½ c. Cheater's Chili Cheese Dip with about 200 calories of whole grain chips

Record nutritional values for your choice of whole grain chips in today's journal. The nutritional values below are for Cheater's Chili Cheese Dip only.

Cal.: 156; Fat: 5.8 g; Protein: 10 g; Sodium: 769 mg; Fiber: 3 g; Carbs.: 16 g; Sugar: 5.4 g; Zinc: 1.9 mg; Calcium: 253 mg; Iron: 0.73 mg; Vit. D: 0 mcg; Vit. B$_{12}$: 0 mcg

Dinner

Vegetarian burritos with ½ c. vegetarian ground beef substitute, ½ medium tomato, ¼ c. shredded lettuce

Cal.: 387.1; Fat: 5.5 g; Protein: 22.85 g; Sodium: 952.7 mg; Fiber: 13 g; Carbs.: 55.55 g; Sugar: 7.3 g; Zinc: 1.85 mg; Calcium: 104.65 mg; Iron: 3.9 mg; Vit. D: 0 mcg; Vit. B$_{12}$: 0 mcg

Sesame Snow Pea Rice Salad

The leftovers from this rice pilaf can be enjoyed chilled the next day as a cold rice salad. **Serves 4**

4 c. cooked rice
2 T. olive or safflower oil
1 T. sesame oil
2 T. soy sauce
3 T. apple cider vinegar
1 t. sugar

1 c. snow peas, chopped
¾ c. baby corn, chopped
3 scallions, chopped
2 T. chopped fresh parsley
½ t. sea salt

1. In a large pot over low heat, combine the rice, olive oil, sesame oil, soy sauce, vinegar, and sugar, stirring well to combine.
2. Add snow peas, baby corn, and scallions, and heat until warmed through and vegetables are lightly cooked, stirring frequently so the rice doesn't burn.
3. While still hot, stir in fresh parsley and season well with sea salt.

Cheater's Chili Cheese Dip

Serves 5

1 (14.7-oz.) can vegetarian chili

1 (8-oz.) container non-dairy cream cheese substitute

Mix together both ingredients until well combined. Heat, if desired, and serve.

Glasses of Water Consumed: _____

Thoughts About Today: _____

_____

_____

What I Ate Today

Time	Food Item	Amount	Calories	Fat	Carbs	Fiber	Protein
TOTAL							

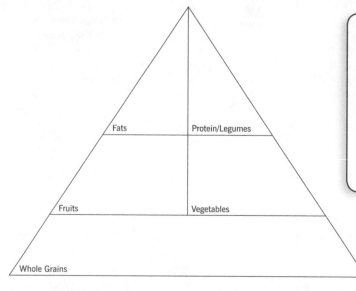

Fats

Protein/Legumes

Fruits

Vegetables

Whole Grains

Eda-What? You're probably familiar with the lightly steamed and salted edamame served as an appetizer at Japanese restaurants, but many grocers sell shelled edamame in the frozen foods section. Edamame, baby green soybeans, are a great source of unprocessed soy protein.

Breakfast

3 Vegan Pancakes with 1 c. fresh strawberries

Cal.: 300.6; Fat: 2.5 g; Protein: 7 g; Sodium: 231.5 mg; Fiber: 6 g; Carbs.: 63.7 g; Sugar: 18.4 g; Zinc: 0.62 mg; Calcium: 282.6 mg; Iron: 3.4 mg; Vit. D: 0 mcg; Vit. B_{12}: 1 mcg

Lunch

1 c. Edamame Salad, 3 oz. baby carrots with 1 T. hummus

Cal.: 560.8; Fat: 29.5 g; Protein: 25.7 g; Sodium: 190.8 mg; Fiber: 14.4 g; Carbs.: 57.1 g; Sugar: 8 g; Zinc: 2.4 mg; Calcium: 1.62 mg; Iron: 9 mg; Vit. D: 0 mcg; Vit. B_{12}: 0 mcg

Snack

½ bagel with 2 T. guacamole, ¼ medium tomato, sliced, 1 oz. pecans

Cal.: 330.53; Fat: 22.65 g; Protein: 8.53 g; Sodium: 146.05 mg; Fiber: 6.33 g; Carbs.: 28.1 g; Sugar: 3.86 g; Zinc: 2.55 mg; Calcium: 64.53 mg; Iron: 3.18 mg; Vit. D: 0 mcg; Vit. B_{12}: 0 mcg

Dinner

1½ c. Spanish Artichoke and Zucchini Paella, 1 c. steamed spinach with 16 g nutritional yeast

Cal.: 282.9; Fat: 4.15 g; Protein: 19.6 g; Sodium: 753.5 mg; Fiber: 13.55 g; Carbs.: 49.2 g; Sugar: 2.12 g; Zinc: 4.69 mg; Calcium: 326 mg; Iron: 10.85 mg; Vit. D: 0 mcg; Vit. B_{12}: 7.8 mcg

Vegan Pancakes

Yields 1 dozen pancakes

1 c. flour
1 T. sugar
1¾ t. baking powder
¼ t. salt
½ banana
1 t. vanilla
1 c. soy milk

1. Mix together flour, sugar, baking powder, and salt in a large bowl.
2. In a separate small bowl, mash banana with a fork. Add vanilla and whisk until smooth. Add soy milk and stir to combine.
3. Add soy milk mixture to the dry ingredients, stirring until combined.
4. Heat a lightly greased frying pan over medium heat. Drop batter about 3 T. at a time and heat until bubbles appear on surface, about 2–3 minutes. Flip and cook other side until lightly golden brown.

Edamame Salad

Serves 4

2 c. frozen shelled edamame, thawed and drained
1 red or yellow bell pepper, diced
¾ c. corn kernels
3 T. chopped fresh cilantro
3 T. olive oil
2 T. red wine vinegar
1 t. soy sauce
1 t. chili powder
2 t. lemon juice

1. Combine edamame, bell pepper, corn, and cilantro in a large bowl.
2. Whisk together olive oil, vinegar, soy sauce, chili powder, and lemon juice. Combine with edamame and chill for at least 1 hour.

Spanish Artichoke and Zucchini Paella

Serves 4

3 cloves garlic, minced
1 yellow onion, diced
1 c. white rice
1 (15-oz.) can diced or crushed tomatoes
1 green bell pepper, chopped
1 red or yellow bell pepper, chopped
½ c. artichoke hearts, chopped
2 zucchinis, sliced
2 c. vegetable broth
1 T. paprika
½ t. turmeric
¾ t. parsley
½ t. salt

1. In a large skillet, heat garlic and onion in olive oil for 3–4 minutes. Add rice, stirring well to coat, and heat for 1 minute.
2. Add tomatoes, bell peppers, artichokes, and zucchini, stirring to combine. Add vegetable broth and remaining ingredients, cover, and simmer for 15–20 minutes, or until rice is done.

Glasses of Water Consumed: _____

Thoughts About Today: _____

_____

_____

What I Ate Today

Time	Food Item	Amount	Calories	Fat	Carbs	Fiber	Protein
TOTAL							

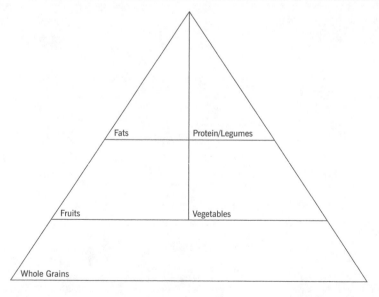

Fats · Protein/Legumes · Fruits · Vegetables · Whole Grains

WEEK 3 IN REVIEW

I feel: _____

_____

_____

_____

My greatest food discovery this week was: _____

_____

_____

_____

This week's biggest vegan challenge was: _____

_____

_____

_____

New food I'd like to try: _____

_____

_____

_____

When I look back at this week, I most want to remember: _____

_____

_____

_____

Nutrition Totals

	Calories	Fat	Carbs	Fiber	Protein
Goal					
Actual					

WEEK 4

By the end of this week, you'll have been vegan for nearly a whole month! This is a great milestone. Are you proud of yourself? You should be! But you're not quite there yet. Behavioral studies suggest that it takes just over two months to establish new daily habits. This week, while things are settling into more of a routine, focus on how far you've come, and take a look back at what got you going in the first place. Your internal motivation and commitment to your goals will be your strength for the next couple of weeks.

Take time to review your original reasons for going vegan. Was it an online video about factory farming that inspired you to eat a more compassionate diet? Rewatch that video this week to keep yourself motivated. Was it an interview with a celebrity touting the miracle health and beauty benefits of a plant-based diet? Reread that interview. Tweet it, post it to Facebook, and keep it handy to keep you motivated, inspired, and educated. Revisit the goals that you wrote down before day one. How are you doing? Is it time to update them again?

After nearly a month of vegan eating, you're likely to have noticed a change in your tastes and preferences. This week, try out some new whole grains as well as more vegan substitutes. Try a few different brands and flavors of vegan cheese to see which you like best, and watch out for hidden milk in the form of casein. As for the grains, check out the bulk bins at your natural-foods store to buy as little or as much as you need and for the best prices.

Breakfast

¾ c. whole grain cereal, 1 c. soy milk

Cal.: 178.33; Fat: 2.92 g; Protein: 6.17 g; Sodium: 267.83 mg; Fiber: 4.6 g; Carbs.: 33.43 g; Sugar: 7.17 g; Zinc: 20 mg; Calcium: 1373.33 mg; Iron: 24.7 mg; Vit. D: 54.7 mcg; Vit. B$_{12}$: 8.51 mcg

Lunch

½ c. Eggless Egg Salad on 2 slices whole grain bread, mixed veggies (½ cucumber, 2 oz. baby carrots, ½ c. broccoli) with 2 T. hummus

Cal.: 436.65; Fat: 17.57 g; Protein: 23.66 g; Sodium: 692.05 mg; Fiber: 12.4 g; Carbs.: 51.87 g; Sugar: 13.32 g; Zinc: 3.32 mg; Calcium: 525.91 mg; Iron: 5.66 mg; Vit. D: 0 mcg; Vit. B$_{12}$: 0 mcg

Snack

One leftover Vegan Pancake (see recipe in Week 3, Sun.) with 1 T. peanut butter, 2 oz. banana chips

Cal.: 474; Fat: 27.47 g; Protein: 8.53 g; Sodium: 83.07 mg; Fiber: 6.4 g; Carbs.: 52.93 g; Sugar: 24.47 g; Zinc: 0.61 mg; Calcium: 96 mg; Iron: 1.73 mg; Vit. D: 0 mcg; Vit. B$_{12}$: 0.33 mcg

Dinner

1½ c. Pumpkin and Lentil Curry with Quinoa

Cal.: 326; Fat: 12 g; Protein: 13 g; Sodium: 17 mg; Fiber: 13 g; Carbs.: 43 g; Sugar: 3.2 g; Zinc: 2.5 mg; Calcium: 67 mg; Iron: 5.9 mg; Vit. D: 0 mcg; Vit. B$_{12}$: 0 mcg

Eggless Egg Salad

Serves 4

1 block firm tofu
1 block silken tofu
½ c. vegan mayonnaise
⅓ c. sweet pickle relish
¾ t. apple cider vinegar
½ stalk celery, diced

2 T. minced onion
1½ T. Dijon mustard
2 T. chopped chives (optional)
2 T. vegetarian bacon bits (optional)
1 t. paprika

1. In a medium-sized bowl, use a fork to mash the tofu together with the rest of the ingredients, except the bacon bits and paprika.
2. Chill for at least 15 minutes before serving to allow flavors to mingle.
3. Garnish with vegetarian bacon bits and paprika just before serving.

Pumpkin and Lentil Curry with Quinoa

Serves 3

1 yellow onion, chopped
2 c. chopped pumpkin or butternut squash
2 T. olive oil
1 T. curry powder
1 t. cumin
2 small red chilies, minced, or ½ t. red pepper flakes
2 whole cloves

3 c. water or vegetable broth
1 c. lentils
2 tomatoes, chopped
8–10 fresh green beans, trimmed and chopped
¾ c. coconut milk
1½ c. cooked quinoa, prepared according to package

1. Sauté onion and pumpkin in olive oil until onion is soft, about 4 minutes. Add curry powder, cumin, chilies, and cloves, and toast for 1 minute, stirring frequently.
2. Reduce heat slightly and add water or vegetable broth and lentils. Cover and cook for about 10–12 minutes, stirring occasionally.
3. Uncover and add tomatoes, green beans, and coconut milk, stirring well to combine. Heat uncovered for 4–5 more minutes, just until tomatoes and beans are cooked.
4. Serve over cooked quinoa.

Date _____ / _____ / _____

Glasses of Water Consumed: _____

Thoughts About Today: _____

_____

_____

What I Ate Today

Time	Food Item	Amount	Calories	Fat	Carbs	Fiber	Protein
TOTAL							

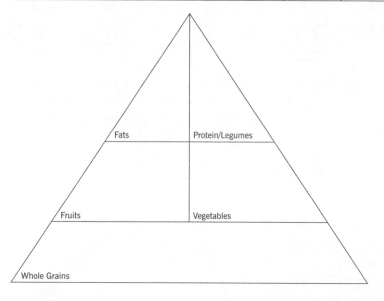

Fats

Protein/Legumes

Fruits

Vegetables

Whole Grains

Tuesday

Breakfast

1 serving Vanilla Date Breakfast Smoothie

Cal.: 530; Fat: 3.8 g; Protein: 9.6 g; Sodium: 75 mg; Fiber: 13 g; Carbs.: 128 g; Sugar: 89 g; Zinc: 0.39 mg; Calcium: 346 mg; Iron: 2.1 mg; Vit. D: 0 mcg; Vit. B$_{12}$: 2.2 mcg

Lunch

1½ c. leftover Pumpkin and Lentil Curry with Quinoa (see recipe in Week 4, Mon.) with ½ c. frozen mixed veggies and 2 T. salad dressing

Record nutritional values for your choice of frozen mixed veggies and salad dressing in today's journal. The nutritional values below are for Pumpkin Lentil Curry with Quinoa alone.

Cal.: 326; Fat: 12 g; Protein: 13 g; Sodium: 17 mg; Fiber: 13 g; Carbs.: 43 g; Sugar: 3.2 g; Zinc: 2.5 mg; Calcium: 67 mg; Iron: 5.9 mg; Vit. D: 0 mcg; Vit. B$_{12}$: 0 mcg

Snack

1 oz. rice cakes with 1 T. almond butter

Cal.: 211; Fat: 10.7 g; Protein: 4.4 g; Sodium: 21.7 mg; Fiber: 1.8 g; Carbs.: 26.1 g; Sugar: 0.2 g; Zinc: 1.3 mg; Calcium: 46.3 mg; Iron: 1 mg; Vit. D: 0 mcg; Vit. B$_{12}$: 0 mcg

Dinner

1 c. Gingered Bok Choy and Tofu Stir-Fry, 1 c. brown rice

Cal.: 610; Fat: 31.8 g; Protein: 35 g; Sodium: 1531.8 mg; Fiber: 7.5 g; Carbs.: 56.8 g; Sugar: 2.7 g; Zinc: 4.4 mg; Calcium: 1135.5 mg; Iron: 6.6 mg; Vit. D: 0 mcg; Vit. B$_{12}$: 0 mcg

Vanilla Date Breakfast Smoothie

Adding dates to a basic soy milk and fruit smoothie adds a blast of unexpected sweetness. Soaking your dates first will help them process a little quicker and results in a smoother consistency. **Serves 1**

4 dates	2 bananas
Water	6–7 ice cubes
¾ c. soy milk	¼ t. vanilla

1. Cover the dates with water and allow to soak for at least 10 minutes. This makes them softer and easier to blend.
2. Discard the soaking water and add the dates and all other ingredients to the blender.
3. Process until smooth; about 1 minute on medium speed.

Gingered Bok Choy and Tofu Stir-Fry

Dark, leafy bok choy is a highly nutritious vegetable that can be found in well-stocked groceries. Keep an eye out for light-green baby bok choy, which are a bit more tender but carry a similar flavor. **Serves 3**

3 T. soy sauce	2 T. olive oil
2 T. lemon or lime juice	1 head bok choy or 3–4
1 T. fresh ginger, minced	small baby bok choys
1 block firm or extra-firm tofu, well pressed	½ t. sugar
	½ t. sesame oil

1. Whisk together soy sauce, lemon or lime juice, and ginger in a shallow pan. Cut tofu into cubes, and marinate for at least one hour. Drain, reserving marinade.
2. In a large skillet or wok, sauté tofu in olive oil for 3–4 minutes.
3. Carefully add reserved marinade, bok choy, and sugar, stirring well to combine.
4. Cook, stirring, for 3–4 more minutes, or until bok choy is done. Drizzle with sesame oil and serve over rice.

Glasses of Water Consumed: _____

Thoughts About Today: _____

_____

_____

What I Ate Today

Time	Food Item	Amount	Calories	Fat	Carbs	Fiber	Protein
TOTAL							

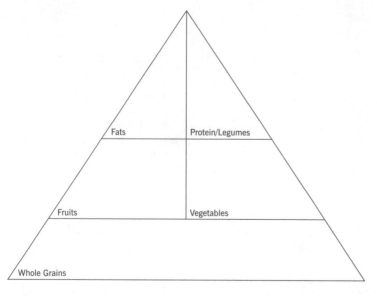

Fats

Protein/Legumes

Fruits

Vegetables

Whole Grains

Wednesday

Breakfast

1 c. soy yogurt with ⅓ c. granola

Cal.: 334; Fat: 12.5 g; Protein: 10.2 g; Sodium: 91.1 mg; Fiber: 4.2 g; Carbs.: 51.2 g; Sugar: 26.7 g; Zinc: 1.2 mg; Calcium: 44.7 mg; Iron: 1.4 mg; Vit. D: 0 mcg; Vit. B$_{12}$: 0 mcg

Lunch

½ c. leftover Gingered Bok Choy and Tofu Stir-Fry (see recipe in Week 4, Tues.), 1 c. brown rice

Cal.: 511; Fat: 24.3 g; Protein: 27.5 g; Sodium: 1151.3 mg; Fiber: 6.5 g; Carbs.: 53.8 g; Sugar: 2.2 g; Zinc: 3.6 mg; Calcium: 856.5 mg; Iron: 5.15 mg; Vit. D: 0 mcg; Vit. B$_{12}$: 0 mcg

Snack

1 c. unsweetened applesauce, 1½ oz. mixed dried fruit (½ oz. raisins, ½ oz. dried cranberries, ½ oz. dried apricots)

Cal.: 221.1; Fat: 0.5 g; Protein: 1.3 g; Sodium: 8.25 mg; Fiber: 5 g; Carbs.: 59 g; Sugar: 47.85 g; Zinc: 0.2 mg; Calcium: 25.95 mg; Iron: 1.25 mg; Vit. D: 0 mcg; Vit. B$_{12}$: 0 mcg

Dinner

1½ c. Bulgur Wheat Tabouli with 2 Easy Falafel Patties and 1 T. tahini

Cal.: 567.2; Fat: 15 g; Protein: 19.4 g; Sodium: 1491.3 mg; Fiber: 14.8 g; Carbs.: 77.2 g; Sugar: 5.39 g; Zinc: 3.7 mg; Calcium: 145.9 mg; Iron: 5 mg; Vit. D: 0 mcg; Vit. B$_{12}$: 0 mcg

Bulgur Wheat Tabouli

Though you'll need to adjust the cooking time, of course, you can try this tabouli recipe with just about any whole grain. Bulgur wheat is traditional, but quinoa, millet, or amaranth would also work. **Serves 4**

1¼ c. boiling water or vegetable broth	½ t. pepper
1 c. bulgur wheat	3 scallions, chopped
3 T. olive oil	½ c. chopped fresh mint
¼ c. lemon juice	½ c. chopped fresh parsley
1 t. garlic powder	1 (15-oz.) can chickpeas, drained (optional)
½ t. sea salt	3 large tomatoes, diced

1. Pour boiling water over bulgur wheat. Cover, and allow to sit for 30 minutes, or until bulgur wheat is soft.
2. Toss bulgur wheat with olive oil, lemon juice, garlic powder, and salt, stirring well to coat. Combine with remaining ingredients, adding in tomatoes last.
3. Allow to chill for at least 1 hour before serving.

Easy Falafel Patties

Health-food stores sell a vegan instant falafel mix, but it's not very much work at all to make your own from scratch. **Serves 4**

1 (15-oz.) can chickpeas, well drained	¾ t. salt
½ onion, minced	Egg substitute for 1 egg
1 T. flour	¼ c. chopped fresh parsley
1 t. cumin	2 T. chopped fresh cilantro (optional)
¾ t. garlic powder	

1. Preheat oven to 375°F.
2. Place chickpeas in a large bowl and mash with a fork until coarsely mashed. Or, pulse in a food processor until chopped.
3. Combine chickpeas with onion, flour, cumin, garlic, salt, and egg substitute, mashing together to combine. Add parsley and cilantro.
4. Shape mixture into 2-inch balls or 1-inch thick patties and bake in oven for 15 minutes, or until crisp. Falafel can also be fried in oil for about 5–6 minutes on each side.

Glasses of Water Consumed: _____

Thoughts About Today: _____

_____

_____

What I Ate Today

Time	Food Item	Amount	Calories	Fat	Carbs	Fiber	Protein
TOTAL							

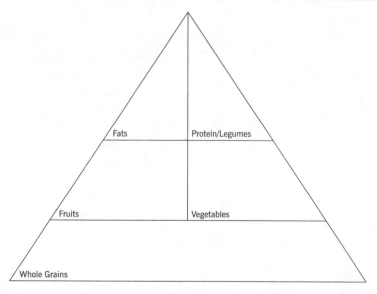

Fats

Protein/Legumes

Fruits

Vegetables

Whole Grains

Thursday

Breakfast

12 oz. Chocolate Peanut Butter Banana Smoothie (see recipe in Week 1, Thurs.), granola bar

Record nutritional values for your choice of granola bar in today's journal. The nutritional stats below are only for the Chocolate Peanut Butter Banana Smoothie.

Cal.: 288; Fat: 11 g; Protein: 10 g; Sodium: 124 mg; Fiber: 7 g; Carbs.: 45 g; Sugar: 20 g; Zinc: 1.1 mg; Calcium: 205 mg; Iron: 1.8 mg; Vit. D: 0 mcg; Vit. B_{12}: 1.5 mcg

Lunch

Leftover Bulgur Wheat Tabouli (see recipe in Week 4, Wed.) and Easy Falafel Patties (see recipe in Week 4, Wed.), 1 c. orange juice

Cal.: 421; Fat: 4.9 g; Protein: 11 g; Sodium: 676 mg; Fiber: 8.8 g; Carbs.: 71 g; Sugar: 27 g; Zinc: 1.7 mg; Calcium: 412 mg; Iron: 1.8 mg; Vit. D: 0 mcg; Vit. B_{12}: 0.41 mcg

Snack

200 calories of whole grain crackers with vegetable salsa

Record nutritional values for your choice of whole grain crackers and vegetable salsa in today's journal.

Dinner

Veggie burger with tomato, lettuce, and avocado, 4 oz. Baked Sweet Potato fries, 1 c. almond milk

Cal.: 521.58; Fat: 23.8 g; Protein: 22.18 g; Sodium: 1051.15 mg; Fiber: 14.03 g; Carbs.: 59.35 g; Sugar: 10.8 g; Zinc: 2 mg; Calcium: 640.38 mg; Iron: 4.53 mg; Vit. D: 0 mcg; Vit. B_{12}: 1.4 mcg

Baked Sweet Potato Fries

Brown sugar adds a sweet touch to these yummy sweet potato fries. If you like your fries with a kick, add some crushed red pepper flakes or a dash of cayenne pepper to the mix. **Serves 3**

2 large sweet potatoes, sliced into fries	½ t. paprika
2 T. olive oil	½ t. brown sugar
¼ t. garlic powder	½ t. chili powder
	¼ t. sea salt

1. Preheat oven to 400°F.
2. Spread sweet potatoes on a large baking sheet and drizzle with olive oil, tossing gently to coat.
3. In a small bowl, combine remaining ingredients. Sprinkle over potatoes, coating evenly and tossing as needed.
4. Bake for 10 minutes, turning once. Taste, and sprinkle with a bit more sea salt, if needed.

The Many Textures of Tofu Freeze firm or extra-firm tofu for an even meatier and chewier texture, which some people prefer, and which makes it even more absorbent. After pressing your tofu, stick it in the freezer until solid and thaw just before using. If you don't use the whole block, cover any leftover bits of uncooked tofu with water in a sealed container and stick it in the fridge.

Thursday

Glasses of Water Consumed: _____

Thoughts About Today: _____

_____

_____

What I Ate Today

Time	Food Item	Amount	Calories	Fat	Carbs	Fiber	Protein
TOTAL							

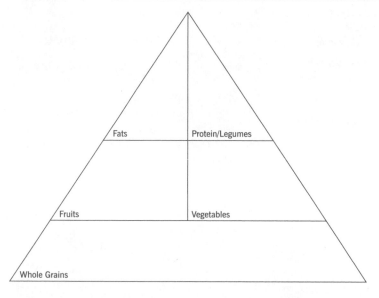

Fats

Protein/Legumes

Fruits

Vegetables

Whole Grains

Friday

Breakfast

¾ c. Maple Cinnamon Breakfast Quinoa, 1 small banana

Cal.: 510.9; **Fat:** 8.7 g; **Protein:** 16.1 g; **Sodium:** 53 mg; **Fiber:** 8 g; **Carbs.:** 98 g; **Sugar:** 24.4 g; **Zinc:** 3.7 mg; **Calcium:** 200.1 mg; **Iron:** 8.9 mg; **Vit. D:** 0 mcg; **Vit. B$_{12}$:** 1 mcg

Snack

1 c. popcorn with 8 g nutritional yeast, 1 c. orange juice

Cal.: 163.1; **Fat:** 0.55 g; **Protein:** 7 g; **Sodium:** 2.8 mg; **Fiber:** 3.2 g; **Carbs.:** 34.7 g; **Sugar:** 22.5 g; **Zinc:** 1.8 mg; **Calcium:** 350.8 mg; **Iron:** 0.55 mg; **Vit. D:** 0 mcg; **Vit. B$_{12}$:** 4.31 mcg

Lunch

Vegan grilled cheese sandwich on 2 slices whole grain bread with 2 (1-oz.) slices vegan cheese, tomato soup (about 150 calories), 1 small apple

Record nutritional values for your choice of tomato soup in today's journal. The nutritional values below are for the vegan grilled cheese sandwich and small apple only.

Cal.: 372.5; **Fat:** 6.8 g; **Protein:** 9.8 g; **Sodium:** 463 mg; **Fiber:** 11 g; **Carbs.:** 73.8 g; **Sugar:** 34.4 g; **Zinc:** 1 mg; **Calcium:** 471 mg; **Iron:** 1.8 mg; **Vit. D:** 0 mcg; **Vit. B$_{12}$:** 0 mcg

Dinner

1 c. Black Bean and Barley Taco Salad

Cal.: 586; **Fat:** 3.2 g; **Protein:** 32 g; **Sodium:** 292 mg; **Fiber:** 24 g; **Carbs.:** 110 g; **Sugar:** 3 g; **Zinc:** 6 mg; **Calcium:** 188 mg; **Iron:** 8.8 mg; **Vit. D:** 0 mcg; **Vit. B$_{12}$:** 0 mcg

Maple Cinnamon Breakfast Quinoa

Quinoa is a filling and healthy breakfast and has more protein than regular oatmeal. This is a deliciously sweet and energizing way to kick off your day. **Serves 2**

1 c. quinoa	½ t. cinnamon
2–2½ c. water	2 T. maple syrup
1 t. vegan margarine	2 T. raisins (optional)
⅔ c. soy milk	2 bananas, sliced (optional)

1. Heat the quinoa and water in a small saucepan and bring to a boil. Reduce to a simmer and allow to cook, covered, for 15 minutes, until liquid is absorbed.
2. Remove from heat and fluff the quinoa with a fork. Cover, and allow to sit for 5 minutes.
3. Stir in the margarine and soy milk, then the remaining ingredients.

Black Bean and Barley Taco Salad

Adding barley to a taco salad gives a bit of a whole grain and fiber boost to this low-fat recipe. **Serves 3**

1 (15-oz.) can black beans, drained	1 c. cooked barley
½ t. cumin	1 head iceberg lettuce, shredded
½ t. oregano	¾ c. salsa
2 T. lime juice	Handful tortilla chips, crumbled
1 t. hot chili sauce (optional)	2 T. vegan Italian dressing (optional)

1. Mash together the beans, cumin, oregano, lime juice, and hot sauce until beans are mostly mashed, then combine with barley.
2. Layer lettuce with beans and barley, and top with salsa and tortilla chips. Drizzle with Italian dressing.

Friday

Glasses of Water Consumed: _____

Thoughts About Today: _____

_____

_____

What I Ate Today

Time	Food Item	Amount	Calories	Fat	Carbs	Fiber	Protein
TOTAL							

Fats · Protein/Legumes · Fruits · Vegetables · Whole Grains

Quinoa for Breakfast If you discover you like eating quinoa for breakfast, try quinoa flakes instead of whole quinoa. The flakes are quicker to cook, like oatmeal, but provide the same protein and amino acids that make quinoa such a great choice for vegans.

Saturday

Breakfast

1 c. instant Cream of Wheat with 1 banana, sliced, 1 c. soy hot chocolate

Cal.: 221.4; Fat: 2.9 g; Protein: 11.5 g; Sodium: 460 mg; Fiber: 5 g; Carbs.: 74.6 g; Sugar: 27.6 g; Zinc: 1.2 mg; Calcium: 459.1 mg; Iron: 13.38 mg; Vit. D: 2.7 mcg; Vit. B$_{12}$: 3 mcg

Lunch

Quesadilla with 2 (1-oz.) slices vegan cheese, 2 oz. chicken substitute, ¼ c. broccoli, and ½ c. black beans

Cal.: 358.5; Fat: 6.57 g; Protein: 17.05 g; Sodium: 44.75 mg; Fiber: 12.43 g; Carbs.: 61.72 g; Sugar: 1.9 g; Zinc: 1.55 mg; Calcium: 379.52 mg; Iron: 4.95 mg; Vit. D: 0 mcg; Vit. B$_{12}$: 0 mcg

Snack

½ bagel with 1 T. hummus, 1 c. orange juice

Cal.: 208; Fat: 1.85 g; Protein: 6.05 g; Sodium: 184.3 mg; Fiber: 1.55 g; Carbs.: 42.6 g; Sugar: 23.45 g; Zinc: 0.85 mg; Calcium: 381.05 mg; Iron: 2.1 mg; Vit. D: 0 mcg; Vit. B$_{12}$: 0.41 mcg

Dinner

½ c. Lentil and Rice Loaf, 1 c. vegan mashed potatoes, 1 ear corn on the cob

Cal.: 551; Fat: 8.2 g; Protein: 23 g; Sodium: 363.8 mg; Fiber: 7.6 g; Carbs.: 102.1 g; Sugar: 4.9 g; Zinc: 4 mg; Calcium: 6.1 mg; Iron: 7.1 mg; Vit. D: 0.8 mcg; Vit. B$_{12}$: 0 mcg

Lentil and Rice Loaf

Made from two of the cheapest ingredients on the planet, this one is a great filler for families on a budget. Use poultry seasoning in place of the individual herbs, if you prefer. **Serves 8**

3 cloves garlic	Egg replacement for 1 egg
1 large onion, diced	½ t. parsley
2 T. oil	½ t. thyme
3½ c. cooked lentils	½ t. oregano
2¼ c. cooked rice	¼ t. sage
⅓ c. + 3 T. ketchup	¾ t. salt
2 T. flour	½ t. black pepper

1. Preheat oven to 350°F.
2. Sauté garlic and onion in oil until onion is soft and clear, about 3–4 minutes.
3. In a large bowl, use a fork or a potato masher to mash the lentils until about ⅔ mashed.
4. Add garlic and onions, rice, ⅓ cup ketchup, and flour and combine well, then add egg replacement and remaining ingredients, mashing to combine.
5. Gently press the mixture into a lightly greased loaf pan. Drizzle the remaining 3 T. ketchup on top.
6. Bake for 60 minutes. Allow to cool at least 10 minutes before serving, as loaf will firm slightly as it cools.

For a Perfect Lentil Loaf . . .

Cook the rice and lentils in vegetable broth and add a bay leaf for maximum flavor. Overcook the lentils a bit, so they'll be soft and mash easily. To avoid a mushy loaf, allow both the rice and lentils to cool completely before making your loaf, as they'll be drier that way. Finally, smother the top with loads of ketchup—that's the best part!

Saturday

Glasses of Water Consumed: _____

Thoughts About Today: _____

_____

_____

What I Ate Today

Time	Food Item	Amount	Calories	Fat	Carbs	Fiber	Protein
TOTAL							

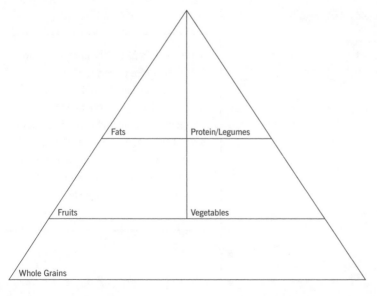

Fats   Protein/Legumes

Fruits   Vegetables

Whole Grains

Sunday

Breakfast

½ c. baked beans, on 2 slices of whole grain toast, 1 small apple

Cal.: 266.6; Fat: 1.9 g; Protein: 9.9 g; Sodium: 591.5 mg; Fiber: 11.5 g; Carbs.: 55.9 g; Sugar: 26.2 g; Zinc: 2.6 mg; Calcium: 75.5 mg; Iron: 3.6 mg; Vit. D: 0 mcg; Vit. B$_{12}$: 0 mcg

Lunch

¾ c. Mediterranean Quinoa Pilaf, 1 c. broccoli

Cal.: 605; Fat: 29.1 g; Protein: 15.3 g; Sodium: 1048.5 mg; Fiber: 10.6 g; Carbs.: 80.6 g; Sugar: 9.1 g; Zinc: 3.3 mg; Calcium: 116 mg; Iron: 9.15 mg; Vit. D: 0 mcg; Vit. B$_{12}$: 0 mcg

Snack

1 c. Edamame, 1 c. almond milk

Cal.: 229; Fat: 12.1 g; Protein: 17.9 g; Sodium: 189.3 mg; Fiber: 9.1 g; Carbs.: 17.8 g; Sugar: 3.4 g; Zinc: 2.1 mg; Calcium: 547.6 mg; Iron: 3.5 mg; Vit. D: 0 mcg; Vit. B$_{12}$: 0 mcg

Dinner

Take-out cheeseless pizza with extra veggies (about 400 calories), side green salad with 2 c. romaine lettuce, 1 tomato, and 1 diced cucumber, 2 T. Goddess Dressing (see recipe in Week 1, Mon.). (Enjoy a night away from the kitchen, and save some leftovers for tomorrow!)

Record nutritional values for your choice of take-out pizza in today's journal. The nutritional values below are for the side green salad and Goddess Dressing only.

Cal.: 203.2; Fat: 12.3 g; Protein: 6.5 g; Sodium: 226.2 mg; Fiber: 6.12 g; Carbs.: 21.9 g; Sugar: 9.76 g; Zinc: 1.58 mg; Calcium: 143.5 mg; Iron: 3.32 mg; Vit. D: 0 mcg; Vit. B$_{12}$: 0 mcg

Mediterranean Quinoa Pilaf

Inspired by the flavors of the Mediterranean, bring this vibrant whole-grain entrée to a vegan potluck and watch it magically disappear. **Serves 4**

1½ c. quinoa
3 c. vegetable broth
3 T. balsamic vinegar
2 T. olive oil
1 T. lemon juice
⅓ t. salt

½ c. sun-dried tomatoes, chopped
½ c. artichoke hearts, chopped
½ c. black or Kalamata olives, sliced

1. In a large skillet or saucepan, bring the quinoa and vegetable broth to a boil, then reduce to a simmer. Cover, and allow quinoa to cook until liquid is absorbed, about 15 minutes. Remove from heat, fluff quinoa with a fork, and allow to stand another 5 minutes.

2. Stir in the balsamic vinegar, olive oil, lemon juice, and salt, then add remaining ingredients, gently tossing to combine. Serve hot.

What's a Pizza Without Cheese?

More and more pizzerias are offering vegan cheese, but cheeseless pizza is more delicious than you might think. When ordering out, fill your pizza with tons of extra toppings—try olives, whole roasted garlic, pineapple, or even broccoli—and sprinkle it with nutritional yeast if you want that cheesy flavor, or try a vegan ranch dressing to dip it in.

Date ____ / ____ / ____

Glasses of Water Consumed: _____

Thoughts About Today: _____

_____

_____

What I Ate Today

Time	Food Item	Amount	Calories	Fat	Carbs	Fiber	Protein
TOTAL							

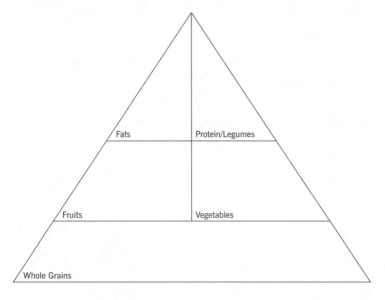

Fats

Protein/Legumes

Fruits

Vegetables

Whole Grains

WEEK 4 IN REVIEW

I feel: _____
_____
_____
_____
_____

My greatest food discovery this week was: _____
_____
_____
_____
_____

This week's biggest vegan challenge was: _____
_____
_____
_____
_____

New food I'd like to try: _____
_____
_____
_____
_____

When I look back at this week, I most want to remember: _____
_____
_____
_____
_____

Nutrition Totals

	Calories	Fat	Carbs	Fiber	Protein
Goal					
Actual					

WEEK 5

Great news! You've been vegan a full month now! Long enough that most of your physical cravings will have subsided by now. Of course, living in a world full of meat eaters, you'll be constantly reminded of what you're not eating, and you may still experience some emotional longing for non-vegan foods, but your tastes have significantly changed by now, and you're probably eating a more varied diet than you ever thought was possible!

If anyone tells you a vegan diet is boring and bland, you'll certainly be proving them wrong this week. It's time to invite friends over to test out your cooking! We'll focus on exploring different palettes of spices and ingredients from around the world, while still keeping the meals simple enough for a busy week.

Two ingredients may be new to you this week: TVP and tempeh. These are both commonly found soy-based meat substitutes that will soon become regular staples in your kitchen. Look for tempeh in the refrigerated section of your regular grocery store, and TVP is usually found among packaged dry foods in natural foods stores. Larger grocers may sell it in the bulk bins, as well. It may look funny, but don't worry, it's delicious when prepared correctly!

Monday

Breakfast

1 c. instant grits with 1 (1-oz.) slice vegan cheese, 1 c. unsweetened applesauce

Cal.: 285; Fat: 2.7 g; Protein: 4.8 g; Sodium: 664.9 mg; Fiber: 3.4 g; Carbs.: 63.6 g; Sugar: 23.1 g; Zinc: 0.3 mg; Calcium: 217.1 mg; Iron: 2.1 mg; Vit. D: 0 mcg; Vit. B$_{12}$: 0 mcg

Lunch

¾ c. leftover Mediterranean Quinoa Pilaf (see recipe in Week 4, Sun.)

Cal.: 556.5; Fat: 28.5 g; Protein: 12 g; Sodium: 1048.5 mg; Fiber: 6 g; Carbs.: 70.5 g; Sugar: 7.2 g; Zinc: 2.7 mg; Calcium: 60 mg; Iron: 8.25 mg; Vit. D: 0 mcg; Vit. B$_{12}$: 0 mcg

Snack

Mixed fruit salad with ½ apple, ½ banana, ½ c. strawberries, and ½ c. pineapple, 1 oz. peanuts

Cal.: 317.25; Fat: 15.35 g; Protein: 9.5 g; Sodium: 92.45 mg; Fiber: 8.35 g; Carbs.: 42.8 g; Sugar: 27 g; Zinc: 1.25 mg; Calcium: 47 mg; Iron: 1.2 mg; Vit. D: 0 mcg; Vit. B$_{12}$: 0 mcg

Dinner

2 c. Ten-Minute Cheater's Chili topped with 1 (1-oz.) slice vegan cheese, ½ c. Crispy Tempeh Fries

Cal.: 609; Fat: 25.6 g; Protein: 40 g; Sodium: 1741 mg; Fiber: 15 g; Carbs.: 71 g; Sugar: 4.47 g; Zinc: 1.67 mg; Calcium: 470 mg; Iron: 9.4 mg; Vit. D: 0 mcg; Vit. B$_{12}$: 0 mcg

Ten-Minute Cheater's Chili

No time? No problem! This is a quick and easy way to get some veggies and protein on the table with no hassle. Instead of veggie burgers, you could toss in a handful of TVP flakes, if you'd like, or any other mock meat you happen to have on hand. **Serves 4**

1 (12-oz.) jar salsa

1 (14-oz.) can diced tomatoes

2 (14-oz.) cans kidney beans or black beans, drained

1½ c. frozen veggies

4 veggie burgers, crumbled (optional)

2 T. chili powder

1 t. cumin

½ c. water

In a large pot, combine all ingredients together. Simmer for 10 minutes, stirring frequently.

Crispy Tempeh Fries

Frying these tempeh sticks twice makes them extra-crispy. **Serves 2**

1 (8-oz.) package tempeh

Water for boiling

½ t. salt

½ t. garlic powder

Oil for frying

Seasoning salt, to taste

1. Slice tempeh into thin strips. Simmer tempeh, covered, in an inch of water for 10 minutes. Drain.
2. While tempeh is still moist, sprinkle with salt and garlic powder.
3. Heat oil and fry tempeh for 5–6 minutes, until crispy and browned. Place tempeh on paper towels and allow to cool for at least 30 minutes.
4. Reheat oil and fry again for another 4–5 minutes. Season lightly with seasoning salt while still warm.

Date ____ / ____ / ____

Glasses of Water Consumed: _____

Thoughts About Today: _____

_____

_____

What I Ate Today

Time	Food Item	Amount	Calories	Fat	Carbs	Fiber	Protein
TOTAL							

Fats

Protein/Legumes

Fruits

Vegetables

Whole Grains

Tempeh 101 Most tempeh recipes will turn out better if your tempeh is simmered in a bit of water or vegetable broth first. This improves the digestibility of the tempeh, softens it up, decreases the cooking time, and, if you add some seasonings such as soy sauce, garlic powder, or some herbs, will increase the flavor, as well.

Tuesday

Breakfast

1 T. almond butter and 1 small banana, sliced, on 2 slices whole wheat bread, soy hot chocolate

Cal.: 429.1; **Fat:** 14 g; **Protein:** 16.5 g; **Sodium:** 317.8 mg; **Fiber:** 8 g; **Carbs.:** 69.1 g; **Sugar:** 30.8 g; **Zinc:** 2.1 mg; **Calcium:** 401.5 mg; **Iron:** 3.38 mg; **Vit. D:** 2.7 mcg; **Vit. B$_{12}$:** 3 mcg

Lunch

Vegetarian baked beans with veggie hot dogs, 1 c. diced pineapple

Cal.: 282.5; **Fat:** 2.7 g; **Protein:** 17.9 g; **Sodium:** 871.7 mg; **Fiber:** 11.3 g; **Carbs.:** 50.6 g; **Sugar:** 25.3 g; **Zinc:** 2.3 mg; **Calcium:** 63.5 mg; **Iron:** 7.2 mg; **Vit. D:** 0 mcg; **Vit. B$_{12}$:** 0 mcg

Snack

½ c. leftover Crispy Tempeh Fries (see recipe in Week 5, Mon.) dipped in ¼ c. Basic Vegetable Marinara (see recipe in Week 1, Mon.)

Cal.: 310.33; **Fat:** 21.33 g; **Protein:** 22.67 g; **Sodium:** 663.33 mg; **Fiber:** 1 g; **Carbs.:** 14.67 g; **Sugar:** 2.5 g; **Zinc:** 1.2 mg; **Calcium:** 137.33 mg; **Iron:** 3.73 mg; **Vit. D:** 0 mcg; **Vit. B$_{12}$:** 0 mcg

Dinner

1½ c. Pineapple Cauliflower Curry with 1 c. brown rice and 1 c. orange juice

Cal.: 633; **Fat:** 19.8 g; **Protein:** 13.7 g; **Sodium:** 285.8 mg; **Fiber:** 11.5 g; **Carbs.:** 105.8 g; **Sugar:** 39.7 g; **Zinc:** 2.9 mg; **Calcium:** 448.5 mg; **Iron:** 3.1 mg; **Vit. D:** 0 mcg; **Vit. B$_{12}$:** 0 mcg

Pineapple Cauliflower Curry

To save time chopping, substitute a bag of mixed frozen veggies or toss in some leftover cooked potatoes to this tropical yellow curry recipe. **Serves 4**

¾ c. vegetable broth

1 c. coconut milk

1½ c. green peas

1 cauliflower, chopped

2 carrots, chopped small

2 t. fresh ginger, minced

3 cloves garlic, minced

2 t. curry powder

½ t. turmeric

1 t. brown sugar

¼ t. salt

¼ t. nutmeg

1 c. diced pineapple

2 T. chopped fresh cilantro (optional)

1. Whisk together the vegetable broth and coconut milk in a large saucepan.
2. Add remaining ingredients except pineapple and cilantro, stirring well to combine. Bring to a slow simmer, cover, and cook for 8–10 minutes, stirring occasionally. Add pineapple and heat for two more minutes.
3. Top with fresh cilantro, if desired, and serve hot over rice or another whole grain.

Make Your Own Nut Butter Nut butters can be very expensive to purchase, but they are so easy to make at home! You can use this method to make just about any kind of nut butter you like. Try making almond, walnut, or macadamia nut butter for a delicious alternative to store-bought peanut butter. Just process the nuts, then add oil and salt to get a taste and consistency that you like. Roasted nuts work best, so heat them in the oven at 400°F for 6–8 minutes or toast them in a dry skillet on the stove-top for a few minutes.

Glasses of Water Consumed: _____

Thoughts About Today: _____

_____

_____

What I Ate Today

Time	Food Item	Amount	Calories	Fat	Carbs	Fiber	Protein
TOTAL							

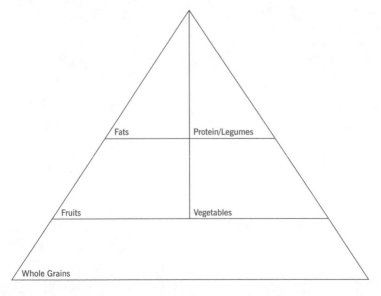

Fats

Protein/Legumes

Fruits

Vegetables

Whole Grains

Wednesday

Breakfast

Cream cheese tortilla wrap with 1 T. vegan cream cheese, ½ small apple, sliced, 1 oz. walnuts, 1 oz. raisins, and ¼ t. cinnamon on a flour tortilla

Cal.: 550.45; Fat: 29.75 g; Protein: 11.9 g; Sodium: 368.65 mg; Fiber: 8 g; Carbs.: 66.9 g; Sugar: 26.25 g; Zinc: 1.05 mg; Calcium: 188.75 mg; Iron: 2.96 mg; Vit. D: 0 mcg; Vit. B$_{12}$: 0 mcg

Lunch

Baked potato with black beans, ¼ c. salsa and 1-oz. slice vegan cheese, 1 c. tomato juice

Cal.: 272.4; Fat: 1 g; Protein: 9.3 g; Sodium: 389.3 mg; Fiber: 5 g; Carbs.: 90.9 g; Sugar: 43.2 g; Zinc: 1 mg; Calcium: 533.4 mg; Iron: 13.3 mg; Vit. D: 0 mcg; Vit. B$_{12}$: 0.41 mcg

Snack

1 (6-inch) pita with 2 T. hummus

Cal.: 215; Fat: 3.5 g; Protein: 7.9 g; Sodium: 435.6 mg; Fiber: 3.1 g; Carbs.: 37.6 g; Sugar: 0.8 g; Zinc: 1.1 mg; Calcium: 63 mg; Iron: 2.4 mg; Vit. D: 0 mcg; Vit. B$_{12}$: 0 mcg

Dinner

1 taco with TVP Taco "Meat," side green salad with 2 c. romaine lettuce, 1 tomato, and 1 diced cucumber, 2 T. Goddess Dressing (see recipe in Week 1, Mon.), 1 c. broccoli with 16 g nutritional yeast

Cal.: 638.4; Fat: 29 g; Protein: 38.7 g; Sodium: 856.8 mg; Fiber: 23.12 g; Carbs.: 65.9 g; Sugar: 13.02 g; Zinc: 13.78 mg; Calcium: 352.1 mg; Iron: 10.32 mg; Vit. D: 0 mcg; Vit. B$_{12}$: 7.8 mcg

TVP Taco "Meat"

Whip up this meaty and economical taco filling in just a few minutes using prepared salsa, and have diners fill their own tacos according to their taste. Nondairy sour cream, fresh tomatoes, shredded lettuce, and extra hot sauce are a must, and find some room on your table for sliced avocados or vegan cheese, if you can. **Serves 6**

2 c. TVP flakes	2 t. chili powder
2 c. hot water	1 t. cumin
1 yellow onion, diced	½ c. salsa
½ red or yellow bell pepper, diced	½ t. hot sauce, or to taste
2 T. olive oil	5–6 flour tortillas or taco shells
½ green bell pepper, diced	

1. Combine TVP with hot water and allow to sit for 5–10 minutes to reconstitute. Drain.
2. In a large skillet, heat onion and bell peppers in olive oil. Add TVP, chili powder, and cumin. Cook, stirring frequently, for 4–5 minutes, or until peppers and onion are soft.
3. Add salsa and hot sauce, stirring to combine. Remove from heat.
4. Wrap TVP mixture in flour tortillas or spoon into taco shells and serve with taco fillings.

Date ___ / ___ / ___

Glasses of Water Consumed: _____

Thoughts About Today: _____

_____

_____

What I Ate Today

Time	Food Item	Amount	Calories	Fat	Carbs	Fiber	Protein
TOTAL							

Fats

Protein/Legumes

Fruits

Vegetables

Whole Grains

Textured Vegetable Protein

TVP is inexpensive and has such a meaty texture that many budget-conscious non-vegetarian cooks use it to stretch their dollar, adding it to homemade burgers and meat loafs. For the best deal, buy it in bulk. TVP is usually found in small crumbles, but some specialty shops also sell it in strips or chunks.

Thursday

Breakfast

¾ c. whole grain cereal, 1 c. soy milk

Cal.: 178.33; Fat: 2.92 g; Protein: 6.17 g; Sodium: 267.83 mg; Fiber: 4.6 g; Carbs.: 33.43 g; Sugar: 7.17 g; Zinc: 20 mg; Calcium: 1373.33 mg; Iron: 24.7 mg; Vit. D: 54.7 mcg; Vit. B$_{12}$: 8.18 mcg

Snack

1 c. soy yogurt with ⅓ c. granola

Cal.: 334; Fat: 12.5 g; Protein: 10.2 g; Sodium: 91.1 mg; Fiber: 4.2 g; Carbs.: 51.2 g; Sugar: 26.7 g; Zinc: 1.2 mg; Calcium: 44.7 mg; Iron: 1.4 mg; Vit. D: 0 mcg; Vit. B$_{12}$: 0 mcg

Lunch

½ c. Tempeh Dill "Chicken" Salad on 2 slices whole grain bread with ¼ tomato, sliced, and ¼ c. iceberg lettuce

Cal.: 356.11; Fat: 5.57 g; Protein: 13.58 g; Sodium: 675.82 mg; Fiber: 10.49 g; Carbs.: 54.95 g; Sugar: 8.23 g; Zinc: 2.03 mg; Calcium: 104.11 mg; Iron: 2.83 mg; Vit. D: 0 mcg; Vit. B$_{12}$: 0 mcg

Dinner

1 c. Thai Tom Kha Coconut Soup with ½ c. brown rice

Cal.: 417; Fat: 18.8 g; Protein: 7.4 g; Sodium: 244.8 mg; Fiber: 5.2 g; Carbs.: 54.8 g; Sugar: 4.5 g; Zinc: 2.1 mg; Calcium: 55.5 mg; Iron: 3.4 mg; Vit. D: 0 mcg; Vit. B$_{12}$: 0 mcg

Tempeh Dill "Chicken" Salad

For curried chicken salad, omit the dill and add ½ t. curry powder and a dash of cayenne and black pepper. **Serves 4**

1 (8-oz.) package tempeh, diced small	1 t. Dijon mustard
Water for boiling	2 T. sweet pickle relish
3 T. vegan mayonnaise	½ c. green peas
2 t. lemon juice	2 stalks celery, diced small
½ t. garlic powder	1 T. chopped fresh dill (optional)

1. Cover tempeh with water and simmer for 10 minutes, until tempeh is soft. Drain and allow to cool completely.
2. Whisk together mayonnaise, lemon juice, garlic powder, mustard, and relish.
3. Combine tempeh, mayonnaise mixture, peas, celery, and dill, and gently toss to combine.
4. Chill for at least one hour before serving to allow flavors to combine.

Thai Tom Kha Coconut Soup

Pair this soup with brown rice for a satisfying meal. Use lime and ginger if you can't find lemongrass or galangal. **Serves 5**

1 (14-oz.) can coconut milk	1–2 small chilies, chopped
2 c. vegetable broth	½ t. red pepper flakes, or to taste
1 T. soy sauce	1 onion, chopped
3 cloves garlic, minced	2 tomatoes, chopped
5 slices fresh ginger or galangal	1 carrot, sliced thin
1 stalk lemongrass, chopped (optional)	½ c. sliced mushrooms, any kind
1 T. lime juice	¼ c. chopped fresh cilantro

1. Combine the coconut milk and vegetable broth over medium-low heat. Add soy sauce, garlic, ginger, lemongrass, lime juice, chilies, and red pepper flakes. Heat, but do not boil.
2. When broth is hot, add onion, tomatoes, carrot, and mushrooms. Cover and cook on low heat for 10–15 minutes.
3. Remove from heat and top with chopped fresh cilantro.

Thursday

Glasses of Water Consumed: _____

Thoughts About Today: _____
_____
_____

What I Ate Today

Time	Food Item	Amount	Calories	Fat	Carbs	Fiber	Protein
TOTAL							

Fats

Protein/Legumes

Fruits

Vegetables

Whole Grains

Got a Big Bunch? Make your fresh herbs last longer by giving them a quick rinse. Then, wrap your lightly damp herbs in a paper towel. Place the paper towel in a zip-lock bag and store in your refrigerator's crisper. They'll keep about ten days this way.

Friday

Breakfast

2 c. Strawberry Protein Smoothie (see recipe in Week 2, Tues.)

Cal.: 204; Fat: 5.5 g; Protein: 10 g; Sodium: 13 mg; Fiber: 3.3 g; Carbs.: 34 g; Sugar: 20 g; Zinc: 1.3 mg; Calcium: 162 mg; Iron: 1.8 mg; Vit. D: 0 mcg; Vit. B$_{12}$: 0 mcg

Lunch

Bean burrito with 1 c. refried beans, ¼ tomato, sliced, and ¼ c. shredded iceberg lettuce

Cal.: 405.53; Fat: 7.93 g; Protein: 18.45 g; Sodium: 1439.8 mg; Fiber: 12.33 g; Carbs.: 67.18 g; Sugar: 1.45 g; Zinc: 1.53 mg; Calcium: 379.25 mg; Iron: 5.08 mg; Vit. D: 0 mcg; Vit. B$_{12}$: 0 mcg

Snack

Mixed fruit salad with ½ apple, ½ banana, ½ c. strawberries, and ½ c. pineapple, granola bar (aim for a fortified bar, with about 150 calories)

Record nutritional values for the granola bar of your choice in today's journal. The nutritional values below are for the mixed fruit salad only.

Cal.: 149.25; Fat: 0.65 g; Protein: 1.7 g; Sodium: 2.85 mg; Fiber: 5.75 g; Carbs.: 38.5 g; Sugar: 25.8 g; Zinc: 0.35 mg; Calcium: 29.9 mg; Iron: 0.8 mg; Vit. D: 0 mcg; Vit. B$_{12}$: 0 mcg

Dinner

1 c. Saucy Chinese Veggies with Seitan or Tempeh with rice noodles, 1 c. orange juice

Cal.: 484; Fat: 11.4 g; Protein: 14.6 g; Sodium: 660.4 mg; Fiber: 3.5 g; Carbs.: 81.8 g; Sugar: 24.4 g; Zinc: 1.1 mg; Calcium: 419 mg; Iron: 2.3 mg; Vit. D: 0 mcg; Vit. B$_{12}$: 0 mcg

Saucy Chinese Veggies with Seitan or Tempeh

This is a simple and basic stir-fry recipe with Asian ingredients and suitable for a main dish. Serve over noodles or rice. **Serves 5**

1½ c. vegetable broth	1 red bell pepper, chopped
3 T. soy sauce	1 c. snow peas
1 T. rice vinegar	½ c. sliced water chestnuts (optional)
1 t. minced ginger	¼ c. sliced bamboo shoots (optional)
1 t. sugar	
1 (8-oz.) block tempeh, cubed, or about 1 c. chopped seitan	2 scallions, sliced
2 T. olive oil	1 T. cornstarch

1. In a small bowl, whisk together the vegetable broth, soy sauce, rice vinegar, ginger, and sugar.
2. In a large skillet, brown the tempeh or seitan in olive oil on all sides, about 3–4 minutes.
3. Add bell pepper, snow peas, water chestnuts, bamboo shoots, and scallions, and heat just until vegetables are almost soft, about 2–3 minutes, stirring constantly.
4. Reduce heat and add vegetable broth mixture. Whisk in cornstarch. Bring to a slow simmer and cook until thickened, stirring to prevent lumps.

That's VEE-gun, Not VAY-gun

Donald Watson, a British farmer, first created the word *vegan* (the beginning and end of "vegetarian," he reasoned) in 1944. He led a mostly quiet life, shunning any fame associated with his revolutionary ideas. At the time of his death at ninety-five years old, he had been vegan for sixty-one years, and vegetarian for more than eighty.

Date ___ / ___ / ___

Glasses of Water Consumed: _____

Thoughts About Today: _____

_____

_____

What I Ate Today

Time	Food Item	Amount	Calories	Fat	Carbs	Fiber	Protein
TOTAL							

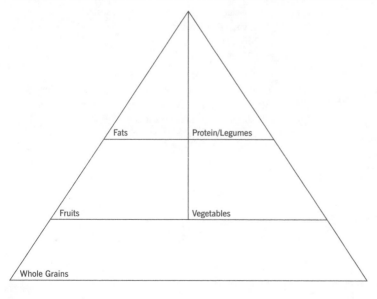

Fats

Protein/Legumes

Fruits

Vegetables

Whole Grains

Saturday

Breakfast

3 oz. Basic Creamy Polenta, 1 vegan sausage patty, 1 c. orange juice

Cal.: 405; Fat: 14 g; Protein: 20 g; Sodium: 1208 mg; Fiber: 5.8 g; Carbs.: 52 g; Sugar: 1.69 g; Zinc: 1.6 mg; Calcium: 24 mg; Iron: 3.94 mg; Vit. D: 0 mcg; Vit. B$_{12}$: 2.28 mcg

Lunch

Vegan Caesar salad with 2 c. romaine lettuce, 3 oz. vegetarian chicken, and store-bought dressing of your choice, 1 small steamed sweet potato, 1 c. orange juice

Record nutritional values for your choice of salad dressing in today's journal. The nutritional values below are for the Vegan Caesar salad, steamed sweet potato, and orange juice only.

Cal.: 292; Fat: 5.2 g; Protein: 12.8 g; Sodium: 213.8 mg; Fiber: 7 g; Carbs.: 50.9 g; Sugar: 26.5 g; Zinc: 0.3 mg; Calcium: 423.3 mg; Iron: 15.9 mg; Vit. D: 0 mcg; Vit. B$_{12}$: 0 mcg

Snack

2 oz. Sugar-Free No-Bake Cocoa Balls

Cal.: 289; Fat: 23 g; Protein: 6 g; Sodium: 5.8 mg; Fiber: 5.8 g; Carbs.: 21 g; Sugar: 12 g; Zinc: 0.57 mg; Calcium: 43 mg; Iron: 1.8 mg; Vit. D: 0 mcg; Vit. B$_{12}$: 0 mcg

Dinner

1 c. Lentil Vegetable Soup, 1 slice whole grain toast, 1 c. oven-roasted butternut squash, 1 c. collard greens sautéed with ½ T. oil, 1 clove garlic, and dash sea salt

Cal.: 597.1; Fat: 12.8 g; Protein: 25.3 g; Sodium: 515.2 mg; Fiber: 27.3 g; Carbs.: 101.4 g; Sugar: 9.62 g; Zinc: 3.38 mg; Calcium: 524.6 mg; Iron: 7.86 mg; Vit. D: 0 mcg; Vit. B$_{12}$: 0 mcg

Basic Creamy Polenta

Serves 4

6½ c. water	1½ t. garlic powder
2 c. cornmeal (polenta)	¼ c. nutritional yeast
3 T. vegan margarine	½ t. salt

1. Bring the water to a boil, then slowly add polenta, stirring to combine.
2. Reduce heat to low, and cook for 20 minutes, stirring frequently. Polenta is done when it is thick and sticky.
3. Stir in margarine, garlic powder, nutritional yeast, and salt.

Sugar-Free No-Bake Cocoa Balls

Serves 5

1 c. chopped pitted dates	¼ c. cocoa powder
Water for soaking	1 T. peanut butter
1 c. walnuts or cashews	¼ c. coconut flakes

1. Cover dates in water and soak for about 10 minutes, until softened. Drain.
2. Process dates, nuts, cocoa powder, peanut butter, and coconut flakes in a food processor until coarse.
3. Shape into balls and chill.

Lentil Vegetable Soup

Serves 4

1 onion, diced	1 c. dry lentils
2 cloves garlic, minced	½ t. dried thyme
2 ribs celery, chopped	¼ t. oregano
1 medium carrot, chopped	2 bay leaves
1 T. olive oil	Salt and pepper, to taste
2 c. water	2 c. spinach
4 c. vegetable broth	Squeeze of lemon juice
2 medium potatoes, chopped	

1. In a large pot, sauté the onion, garlic, celery, and carrot in olive oil for 4–5 minutes, until onion is soft. Reduce heat and add remaining ingredients, except for spinach and lemon juice.
2. Bring to a slow simmer. Cover and heat until lentils are cooked through, about 45 minutes. Stir in spinach leaves and heat another five minutes, until spinach has wilted.
3. Remove bay leaves and drizzle with a generous squeeze of fresh lemon juice just before serving.

Date ____ / ____ / ____

Glasses of Water Consumed: _____

Thoughts About Today: _____

_____

_____

What I Ate Today

Time	Food Item	Amount	Calories	Fat	Carbs	Fiber	Protein
TOTAL							

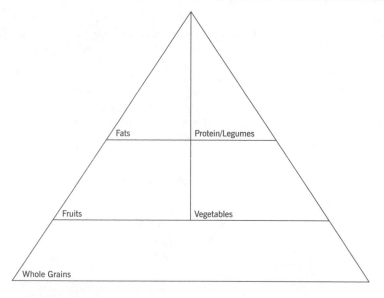

Sunday

Breakfast

1 bagel with 1 T. peanut butter, 1 c. soy milk

Cal.: 336; Fat: 13.4 g; Protein: 17.7 g; Sodium: 287 mg; Fiber: 4.3 g; Carbs.: 37 g; Sugar: 4.9 g; Zinc: 1.1 mg; Calcium: 130.7 mg; Iron: 4.8 mg; Vit. D: 3 mcg; Vit. B_{12}: 0.36 mcg

Snack

1 c. Crispy Baked Kale Chips, 2 oz. cashews

Cal.: 488; Fat: 33.9 g; Protein: 17.9 g; Sodium: 620.8 mg; Fiber: 6.2 g; Carbs.: 40.4 g; Sugar: 3.4 g; Zinc: 3.2 mg; Calcium: 312.8 mg; Iron: 8.3 mg; Vit. D: 0 mcg; Vit. B_{12}: 0.41 mcg

Lunch

1 c. leftover Lentil Vegetable Soup (see recipe in Week 5, Sat.), 1 slice whole grain toast, 1 c. orange juice

Cal.: 485.1; Fat: 4.8 g; Protein: 19.5 g; Sodium: 169 mg; Fiber: 18.9 g; Carbs.: 90.3 g; Sugar: 26.5 g; Zinc: 2.7 mg; Calcium: 446.6 mg; Iron: 6 mg; Vit. D: 0 mcg; Vit. B_{12}: 0 mcg

Dinner

1 c. Cheesy Macaroni and "Hamburger" Casserole, sautéed zucchini

Cal.: 348.8; Fat: 12.1 g; Protein: 19.2 g; Sodium: 877.4 mg; Fiber: 7.3 g; Carbs.: 42.1 g; Sugar: 5.5 g; Zinc: 2 mg; Calcium: 190.4 mg; Iron: 3.6 mg; Vit. D: 0 mcg; Vit. B_{12}: 1.8 mcg

Crispy Baked Kale Chips

Serves 1

1 large bunch of kale
2 t. olive oil
½ t. garlic salt
1 t. nutritional yeast

1. Preheat oven to 350°F.
2. Chop kale into bite-sized pieces and place in a large bowl. Gently toss together with olive oil and garlic salt.
3. Arrange kale in a single layer on a baking sheet and sprinkle well with nutritional yeast. Bake for 20–25 minutes, until nicely crisped.

Cheesy Macaroni and "Hamburger" Casserole

Serves 5

1 (12-oz.) bag macaroni noodles
4 veggie burgers, thawed and crumbled, or 1 (12-oz.) package vegetarian beef crumbles
1 tomato, diced
1 T. olive oil
1 t. chili powder
1 c. soy milk
2 T. vegan margarine
2 T. flour
1 t. garlic powder
1 t. onion powder
¼ c. nutritional yeast
Salt and pepper, to taste

1. Prepare macaroni noodles according to package instructions.
2. Sauté the veggie burgers and tomato in oil until "hamburger" is lightly browned, and season with chili powder.
3. In a separate small skillet, melt together the soy milk and margarine over low heat until well mixed. Stir in flour and heat until thickened, then stir in garlic powder, onion powder, and nutritional yeast and remove from heat.
4. Combine macaroni, veggie burgers, tomato, and sauce, gently tossing to coat.
5. Season generously with salt and pepper, and allow to cool slightly before serving to allow ingredients to combine together.

Sunday

Glasses of Water Consumed: _____

Thoughts About Today: _____

_____

_____

What I Ate Today

Time	Food Item	Amount	Calories	Fat	Carbs	Fiber	Protein
TOTAL							

Fats

Protein/Legumes

Fruits

Vegetables

Whole Grains

Mock Ground Beef Vegetarian ground beef is surprisingly tasty. Use it the same way you would use regular ground beef. Brown it in a bit of oil in a sauté pan and add it to casseroles, pasta sauces, or use as an enchilada or burrito filling. If you have some left over, fry it up and add it to tomorrow's breakfast or dinner.

WEEK 5 IN REVIEW

I feel: _____

_____

_____

_____

My greatest food discovery this week was: _____

_____

_____

_____

This week's biggest vegan challenge was: _____

_____

_____

_____

New food I'd like to try: _____

_____

_____

_____

When I look back at this week, I most want to remember: ___

_____

_____

_____

Nutrition Totals

	Calories	Fat	Carbs	Fiber	Protein
Goal					
Actual					

WEEK 6

By now, your body is mostly done adjusting to your new diet, and you probably haven't been experiencing any withdrawal symptoms for a while. In short, you should be feeling great this week! Your body is getting used to this new way of eating, and you could probably find your way around the grocery store (and your kitchen) in the dark.

If you've never tried seitan, or tried making it yourself, now's your chance. When made from scratch, seitan is the most affordable of all the meat substitutes. It's available store-bought, but making it at home will help your pocketbook immensely. Tofu, tempeh, seitan, and other store-bought mock meats are largely interchangeable, so if you find you like one more than the other, feel free to change it up. They're all great sources of protein. Before you decide that you don't like one of these substitutes, be sure to try it not just once, but twice, two different ways. Look for store-bought seitan (also called wheat gluten) in the refrigerated section of your natural foods store, and avoid the canned kind—it's a bit slimy.

The menu plans call for a bit of experimentation with vegan baking this week and next, so make sure you've got a good egg substitute on hand. If you enjoy baking and don't want to stop with just banana bread and muffins, try a homemade batch of vegan cookies!

Monday

Breakfast

1 c. Chili Masala Tofu Scramble (see recipe in Week 2, Sat.), 1 c. fresh strawberries

Cal.: 362.1; Fat: 21.5 g; Protein: 22.75 g; Sodium: 396.75 mg; Fiber: 7.05 g; Carbs.: 23.7 g; Sugar: 8.9 g; Zinc: 2.9 mg; Calcium: 868.05 mg; Iron: 5.475 mg; Vit. D: 0 mcg; Vit. B$_{12}$: 0 mcg

Lunch

Hummus and roasted red pepper sandwich with 2 T. hummus, 1 oz. roasted red pepper, and ½ c. sprouts, green salad, 2 oz. cashews

Cal.: 608; Fat: 28.2 g; Protein: 21.9 g; Sodium: 395.6 mg; Fiber: 8.4 g; Carbs.: 75.8 g; Sugar: 31.7 g; Zinc: 4.3 mg; Calcium: 429.7 mg; Iron: 6.6 mg; Vit. D: 0 mcg; Vit. B$_{12}$: 0.41 mcg

Snack

200 calories of whole grain chips with ½ c. salsa, 1 small apple

Record nutritional values for your choice of whole grain chips and salsa in today's journal. The nutritional stats below are for a small apple only.

Cal.: 77.5; Fat: 0.3 g; Protein: 0.4 g; Sodium: 1.5 mg; Fiber: 3.6 g; Carbs.: 20.6 g; Sugar: 15.5 g; Zinc: 0.1 mg; Calcium: 8.9 mg; Iron: 0.2 mg; Vit. D: 0 mcg; Vit. B$_{12}$: 0 mcg

Dinner

1 c. Breaded Eggplant "Parmesan"

Cal.: 291; Fat: 3.7 g; Protein: 12 g; Sodium: 1210 mg; Fiber: 5.3 g; Carbs.: 52 g; Sugar: 10 g; Zinc: 1.5 mg; Calcium: 101 mg; Iron: 3.8 mg; Vit. D: 0 mcg; Vit. B$_{12}$: 0.14 mcg

Breaded Eggplant "Parmesan"

Slowly baking these breaded eggplant cutlets brings out the best flavor, but they can also be pan-fried in a bit of oil. **Serves 4**

1 medium eggplant	1½ c. bread crumbs
½ t. salt	2 T. Italian seasonings
¾ c. flour	¼ c. nutritional yeast
1 t. garlic powder	1½ c. Basic Vegetable
⅔ c. soy milk	Marinara (see recipe in
Egg replacement for 2 eggs	Week 1, Mon.)

1. Slice eggplant into ¾-inch-thick slices and sprinkle with salt. Allow to sit for 10 minutes. Gently pat dry to remove extra moisture.
2. In a shallow bowl or pie tin, combine flour and garlic powder. In a separate bowl, whisk together the soy milk and egg replacement. In a third bowl, combine the bread crumbs, Italian seasonings, and nutritional yeast.
3. Coat each eggplant slice with flour, then carefully dip in the soy milk mixture, then coat with the bread crumb mixture and place in a lightly greased casserole dish.
4. Bake for 20–25 minutes, then top with marinara sauce, and return to oven until sauce is hot, about 5 minutes.

Roasted Red Peppers Sure, you can buy them from a jar, but it's also easy to roast your own. Here's how: Fire up your oven to 450°F (or use the broiler setting) and drizzle a few whole peppers with olive oil. Bake for 30 minutes, turning over once. Direct heat will also work, if you have a gas stove. Hold the peppers with tongs over the flame until lightly charred. Once they're cool, removing the skin is optional. Add your roasted red peppers to homemade hummus, sandwiches and wraps, pasta sauces, and salads for a gourmet touch.

Glasses of Water Consumed: _____

Thoughts About Today: _____

_____

_____

What I Ate Today

Time	Food Item	Amount	Calories	Fat	Carbs	Fiber	Protein
TOTAL							

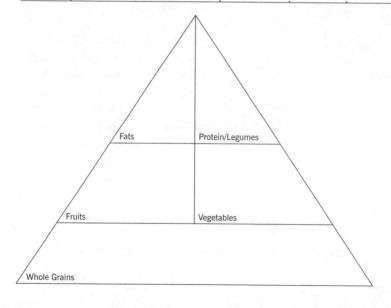

Tuesday

Breakfast

Flour tortilla breakfast wrap with 1 T. almond butter and ⅓ c. granola, 1 c. orange juice

Cal.: 529.9; Fat: 15.4 g; Protein: 16.7 g; Sodium: 416.1 mg; Fiber: 7.3 g; Carbs.: 91.6 g; Sugar: 35.1 g; Zinc: 2 mg; Calcium: 439.2 mg; Iron: 3.78 mg; Vit. D: 2.7 mcg; Vit. B$_{12}$: 3 mcg

Lunch

1 c. leftover Breaded Eggplant "Parmesan" (see recipe in Week 6, Mon.), Greek spinach salad with 2 c. fresh spinach, 1 medium tomato, ½ red bell pepper, 2 T. black olives, ¼ c. chopped artichoke hearts, and 2 T. Goddess Dressing (see recipe in Week 1, Mon.)

Cal.: 494; Fat: 18.3 g; Protein: 17.4 g; Sodium: 1605 mg; Fiber: 10.42 g; Carbs.: 69.2 g; Sugar: 14.36 g; Zinc: 2.08 mg; Calcium: 224 mg; Iron: 90.2 mg; Vit. D: 0 mcg; Vit. B$_{12}$: 0.14 mcg

Snack

Mixed veggies (½ cucumber, 2 oz. baby carrots, ½ c. broccoli) with 2 T. hummus, 1 small banana

Cal.: 206.82; Fat: 3.62 g; Protein: 6.48 g; Sodium: 190.5 mg; Fiber: 9.12 g; Carbs.: 42.47 g; Sugar: 18.52 g; Zinc: 1.47 mg; Calcium: 86.73 mg; Iron: 2.48 mg; Vit. D: 0 mcg; Vit. B$_{12}$: 0 mcg

Dinner

5 oz. Seitan Barbecue "Meat," 1 potato, 1 ear corn on the cob with 16 g nutritional yeast

Cal.: 549; Fat: 18.1 g; Protein: 29 g; Sodium: 450 mg; Fiber: 7.62 g; Carbs.: 79.1 g; Sugar: 4.6 g; Zinc: 5.16 mg; Calcium: 110.1 mg; Iron: 5.5 mg; Vit. D: 0 mcg; Vit. B$_{12}$: 7.8 mcg

Seitan Barbecue "Meat"

Sooner or later, all vegans discover the magically delicious combination of seitan and barbecue sauce in some variation of this classic favorite. **Serves 6**

1 (12-oz.) package prepared seitan, chopped into thin strips (about 2 c.)

1 large onion, chopped

3 cloves garlic, minced

2 T. oil

1 c. barbecue sauce

2 T. water

1. Heat seitan, onion, and garlic in oil, stirring frequently, until onion is just soft and seitan is lightly browned.
2. Reduce heat to medium low and stir in barbecue sauce and water. Allow to simmer, stirring to coat seitan, until most of the liquid has been absorbed, about 10 minutes.

Save the Leftovers for Lunch Tomorrow Piled on top of sourdough along with some vegan mayonnaise, lettuce, and tomato, thinly sliced seitan always makes a perfect sandwich. Melt some vegan cheese for a simple Philly "cheese steak"–style sandwich, or pile on the vegan Thousand Island and sauerkraut for a seitan Reuben. Seitan is also great grilled, so you can also try grilling tonight's seitan instead of pan-frying it.

Tuesday

Glasses of Water Consumed: _____

Thoughts About Today: _____

_____

_____

What I Ate Today

Time	Food Item	Amount	Calories	Fat	Carbs	Fiber	Protein
TOTAL							

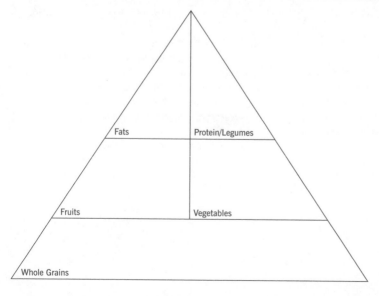

Fats

Protein/Legumes

Fruits

Vegetables

Whole Grains

Wednesday

Breakfast

Oatmeal breakfast bowl with 1 oz. almonds, 1 small banana, and 2 t. maple syrup, soy hot chocolate

Cal.: 535.83; Fat: 19.4 g; Protein: 18 g; Sodium: 97.5 mg; Fiber: 740 g; Carbs.: 11 g; Sugar: 37.99 g; Zinc: 2.25 mg; Calcium: 387.93 mg; Iron: 3.34 mg; Vit. D: 2.7 mcg; Vit. B$_{12}$: 3 mcg

Lunch

5 oz. leftover Seitan Barbecue "Meat" (see recipe in Week 6, Tues.) on two slices of whole wheat bread, with ¼ tomato, sliced ¼ c. shredded iceberg lettuce, and 1 T. vegan mayonnaise, 1 small apple

Cal.: 436.7; Fat: 16.5 g; Protein: 20.4 g; Sodium: 623.5 mg; Fiber: 8.02 g; Carbs.: 56.1 g; Sugar: 20.9 g; Zinc: 1.66 mg; Calcium: 147.1 mg; Iron: 4 mg; Vit. D: 0 mcg; Vit. B$_{12}$: 0 mcg

Snack

½ bagel topped with 2 T. guacamole

Cal.: 132; Fat: 2.4 g; Protein: 5.65 g; Sodium: 144.5 mg; Fiber: 3.25 g; Carbs.: 23 g; Sugar: 1.95 g; Zinc: 1.15 mg; Calcium: 41.85 mg; Iron: 2.4 mg; Vit. D: 0 mcg; Vit. B$_{12}$: 0 mcg

Dinner

1 patty Easy Black Bean Burgers, 2 oz. Breaded Baked Zucchini Chips, 1 c. orange juice

Cal.: 478; Fat: 2.6 g; Protein: 21.1 g; Sodium: 566 mg; Fiber: 11 g; Carbs.: 93 g; Sugar: 24.9 g; Zinc: 2.98 mg; Calcium: 510 mg; Iron: 5.2 mg; Vit. D: 2.25 mcg; Vit. B$_{12}$: 0.29 mcg

Easy Black Bean Burgers

Veggie burgers are notorious for falling apart. If you're sick of crumbly burgers, try this simple method for making black bean patties. It's 100 percent guaranteed to stick together. **Yields 6 patties**

1 (15-oz.) can black beans, drained	2 t. parsley
3 T. minced onions	1 t. chili powder
1 t. salt	⅔ c. flour
1½ t. garlic powder	Oil for pan-frying

1. Process the black beans in a blender or food processor until halfway mashed, or mash with a fork.
2. Add minced onions, salt, garlic powder, parsley, and chili powder, and mash to combine.
3. Add flour, a bit at time, again mashing together to combine. You may need a little bit more or less than ⅔ cup. Beans should stick together completely.
4. Form into patties and pan-fry in a bit of oil for 2–3 minutes on each side. Patties will appear to be done on the outside while still a bit mushy on the inside, so fry them a few minutes longer than you think they need.

Breaded Baked Zucchini Chips

Serves 4

¾ c. fine bread crumbs	¼–⅓ c. soy milk
½ t. Italian seasoning blend	2 zucchini, sliced into ½-inch-thick rounds
½ t. garlic powder	
¼ t. salt	

1. Preheat oven to 475°F and lightly grease a baking sheet.
2. In a large bowl, combine bread crumbs, Italian seasoning, garlic powder, and salt. Place soy milk in a separate small bowl.
3. Gently dip each slice of zucchini into the soy milk, then coat well with bread crumb mix. Arrange breaded zucchini slices on a single layer on baking tray, then bake for 5–10 minutes, or until lightly crisped. Turn zucchini chips over, then bake for another 5 minutes.

Wednesday

Glasses of Water Consumed: _____

Thoughts About Today: _____

_____

_____

What I Ate Today

Time	Food Item	Amount	Calories	Fat	Carbs	Fiber	Protein
TOTAL							

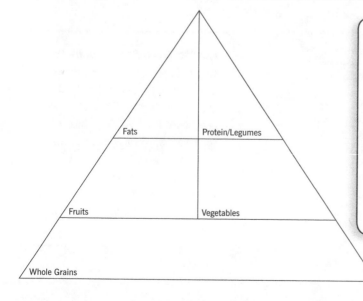

Veggie Burger Tips If you have trouble with your homemade veggie burgers crumbling, try adding egg replacement to bind the ingredients, then chill the mixture before forming into patties. Veggie burger patties can be grilled, baked, or pan-fried, but they do tend to dry out a bit in the oven. Not a problem, though—just smother with extra ketchup!

Thursday

Breakfast

1 c. Pumpkin Protein Smoothie (see recipe in Week 3, Thurs.), 1 small banana, 1 oz. cashews

Cal.: 371.9; Fat: 15.4 g; Protein: 11.6 g; Sodium: 67.4 mg; Fiber: 5.5 g; Carbs.: 53.3 g; Sugar: 22.8 g; Zinc: 2.56 mg; Calcium: 260.5 mg; Iron: 2.2 mg; Vit. D: 1.4 mcg; Vit. B$_{12}$: 1.5 mcg

Lunch

Peanut butter and jelly sandwich on whole grain bread with 1 T. peanut butter and 1 T. sugar-free jam, 1 small apple

Cal.: 357.7; Fat: 10.5 g; Protein: 11.4 g; Sodium: 228.5 mg; Fiber: 8.4 g; Carbs.: 56.2 g; Sugar: 27.5 g; Zinc: 0.9 mg; Calcium: 62.1 mg; Iron: 2.1 mg; Vit. D: 0 mcg; Vit. B$_{12}$: 0 mcg

Snack

2 oz. leftover Breaded Baked Zucchini Chips (see recipe in Week 6, Wed.)

Cal.: 104; Fat: 1.6 g; Protein: 4.1 g; Sodium: 352 mg; Fiber: 1.3 g; Carbs.: 18 g; Sugar: 1.5 g; Zinc: 0.38 mg; Calcium: 81 mg; Iron: 3 mg; Vit. D: 0 mcg; Vit. B$_{12}$: 0 mcg

Dinner

2 Fresh Mint Spring Rolls, ½ c. Baked Teriyaki Tofu Cubes (see recipe in Week 3, Fri.)

Cal.: 468; Fat: 8.5 g; Protein: 22 g; Sodium: 1752 mg; Fiber: 4.7 g; Carbs.: 79.3 g; Sugar: 17.3 g; Zinc: 3.13 mg; Calcium: 566 mg; Iron: 4.1 mg; Vit. D: 0 mcg; Vit. B$_{12}$: 0 mcg

Fresh Mint Spring Rolls

Serves 5

1 (3-oz.) package clear bean thread noodles

1 c. hot water

1 T. soy sauce

½ t. powdered ginger

1 t. sesame oil

¼ c. shiitake mushrooms, diced

1 carrot, grated

1 cucumber, sliced thin

½ head green leaf lettuce, chopped

1 bunch fresh mint

10–12 spring roll wrappers

Warm water

1. Break noodles in half to make smaller pieces, then submerge in 1 cup hot water until soft, about 6–7 minutes. Drain.
2. In a large bowl, toss together the hot noodles with the soy sauce, ginger, sesame oil, mushrooms, and carrot, tossing well to combine.
3. In a large shallow pan, carefully submerge spring roll wrappers, one at a time, in warm water until just barely soft. Remove from water and place a bit of lettuce in the center of the wrapper. Add about 2 T. of noodle mixture, a few slices of cucumber, and place 2–3 mint leaves on top.
4. Fold the bottom of the wrapper over the filling, fold in each side, then roll.

How to Wrap Spring Rolls Wrapping spring rolls is a balance between getting them tight enough to hold together, but not so tight the thin wrappers break! It's like riding a bike: once you've got it, you've got it, and then spring rolls can be very quick and fun to make. Dip them in store-bought sweet chili sauce, spicy sriracha sauce, Japanese salad dressing, or Chinese hoisin sauce.

Date ___ / ___ / ___

Glasses of Water Consumed: _____

Thoughts About Today: _____

_____

_____

What I Ate Today

Time	Food Item	Amount	Calories	Fat	Carbs	Fiber	Protein
TOTAL							

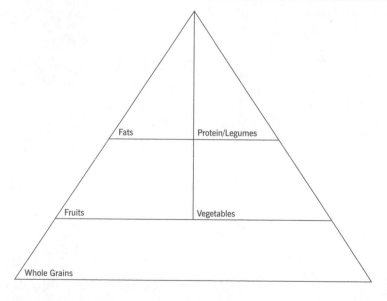

Friday

Breakfast

1 c. whole grain cereal with ½ c. soy milk

Cal.: 178.33; Fat: 2.92 g; Protein: 6.17 g; Sodium: 267.83 mg; Fiber: 4.6 g; Carbs.: 33.43 g; Sugar: 7.17 g; Zinc: 20 mg; Calcium: 1373.33 mg; Iron: 247.7 mg; Vit. D: 54.7 mcg; Vit. B$_{12}$: 8.18 mcg

Lunch

1 c. cooked quinoa with 1 c. spinach and zucchini

Cal.: 257.7; Fat: 3.8 g; Protein: 10.2 g; Sodium: 42.1 mg; Fiber: 8.4 g; Carbs.: 47.6 g; Sugar: 3.1 g; Zinc: 2.5 mg; Calcium: 84.6 mg; Iron: 4.2 mg; Vit. D: 0 mcg; Vit. B$_{12}$: 0 mcg

Snack

1 c. edamame

Cal.: 189; Fat: 8.1 g; Protein: 16.9 g; Sodium: 9.3 mg; Fiber: 8.1 g; Carbs.: 15.8 g; Sugar: 3.4 g; Zinc: 2.1 mg; Calcium: 97.6 mg; Iron: 3.5 mg; Vit. D: 0 mcg; Vit. B$_{12}$: 0 mcg

Dinner

5 oz. Tofu "Chicken" Nuggets, 1 ear corn on the cob, 1 medium sweet potato

Cal.: 463; Fat: 11.8 g; Protein: 25.7 g; Sodium: 883 mg; Fiber: 5.2 g; Carbs.: 71.3 g; Sugar: 4.76 g; Zinc: 3.3 mg; Calcium: 639.2 mg; Iron: 5.8 mg; Vit. D: 0 mcg; Vit. B$_{12}$: 0.32 mcg

Tofu "Chicken" Nuggets

Serves 4

¼ c. soy milk
2 T. mustard
3 T. nutritional yeast
½ c. bread crumbs
½ c. flour
1 t. poultry seasoning
1 t. garlic powder

1 t. onion powder
½ t. salt
¼ t. pepper
1 block firm or extra-firm tofu, sliced into thin strips
Oil for frying (optional)

1. In a large shallow pan, whisk together the soy milk, mustard, and nutritional yeast. In a separate bowl, combine the bread crumbs with the flour, poultry seasoning, garlic powder, onion powder, salt, and pepper.
2. Coat each piece of tofu with the soy milk mixture, then coat well in bread crumbs and flour mixture.
3. Fry in hot oil until lightly golden browned, about 3–4 minutes on each side, or bake in 375°F oven for 20 minutes, turning over once.

Date ____ / ____ / ____

Glasses of Water Consumed: _____

Thoughts About Today: _____

_____

_____

What I Ate Today

Time	Food Item	Amount	Calories	Fat	Carbs	Fiber	Protein
TOTAL							

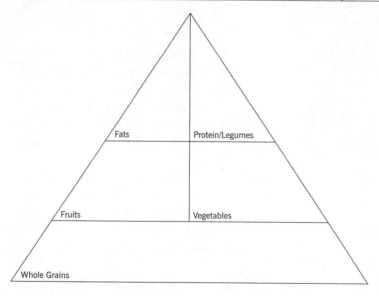

Saturday

Breakfast

2 oz. Basic Creamy Polenta (see recipe in Week 5, Sat.) with 2 (1-oz.) slices vegan cheese, ¼ c. black beans, and 2 T. vegetable salsa

Record nutritional values for your choice of vegetable salsa in today's journal. The nutrition values below are for Basic Creamy Polenta with vegan cheese and black beans only.

Cal.: 395.5; Fat: 6.45 g; Protein: 14.2 g; Sodium: 260.45 mg; Fiber: 11.5 g; Carbs.: 73.4 g; Sugar: 0.4 g; Zinc: 1.95 mg; Calcium: 426.6 mg; Iron: 3.8 mg; Vit. D: 0 mcg; Vit. B$_{12}$: 0 mcg

Lunch

1½ c. Italian White Bean and Fresh Herb Salad (see recipe in Week 1, Fri.), 1 apple

Cal.: 337.5; Fat: 10.8 g; Protein: 15 g; Sodium: 124.5 mg; Fiber: 11.4 g; Carbs.: 49.5 g; Sugar: 3.45 g; Zinc: 1.95 mg; Calcium: 165 mg; Iron: 6 mg; Vit. D: 0 mcg; Vit. B$_{12}$: 0 mcg

Snack

Mixed fruit salad with ½ apple, ½ banana, ½ c. strawberries, and ½ c. pineapple, granola bar (aim for a fortified bar, with about 150 calories)

Record nutritional values for your choice of granola bar in today's journal. If you decide to substitute fruit, make sure to record those values, too. The nutritional values below are for the mixed fruit salad as stated above only.

Cal.: 149.25; Fat: 0.65 g; Protein: 1.7 g; Sodium: 2.85 mg; Fiber: 5.75 g; Carbs.: 38.5 g; Sugar: 25.8 g; Zinc: 0.35 mg; Calcium: 29.9 mg; Iron: 0.8 mg; Vit. D: 0 mcg; Vit. B$_{12}$: 0 mcg

Dinner

5 oz. Classic Fettuccine Alfredo, ½ lb. collard greens sautéed with ½ T. oil, 1 clove garlic, and dash sea salt

Cal.: 494; Fat: 26.8 g; Protein: 20 g; Sodium: 1349 mg; Fiber: 10.4 g; Carbs.: 48.6 g; Sugar: 2.42 g; Zinc: 3.08 mg; Calcium: 407 mg; Iron: 3.66 mg; Vit. D: 0 mcg; Vit. B$_{12}$: 0.18 mcg

Classic Fettuccine Alfredo

Serves 4

½ c. raw cashews
1¼ c. water
1 T. miso
2 T. lemon juice
2 T. tahini
¼ c. diced onion

1 t. garlic
½ t. salt
¼ c. nutritional yeast
2 T. olive or safflower oil
1 (12-oz.) package fettuccine, cooked

1. Blend together the cashews and water until completely smooth and creamy, about 90 seconds.
2. Add remaining ingredients, except oil and fettuccine noodles, and puree until smooth. Slowly add oil until thick and oil is emulsified.
3. Heat in a saucepan over low heat for 4–5 minutes, stirring frequently. Serve over cooked fettuccine noodles.

Vegan Cheese Sauces Most vegan Alfredo recipes start with a roux of margarine and soy milk, but this one uses cashew cream instead for a sensually decadent white sauce. The nutritional yeast is what adds the satisfying cheesy flavor in this recipe, so use it generously! Go ahead and lick the spoons; nobody's watching. Make a double batch of the sauce tonight to use in tomorrow night's gourmet lasagna.

Glasses of Water Consumed: _____

Thoughts About Today: _____

_____

_____

What I Ate Today

Time	Food Item	Amount	Calories	Fat	Carbs	Fiber	Protein
TOTAL							

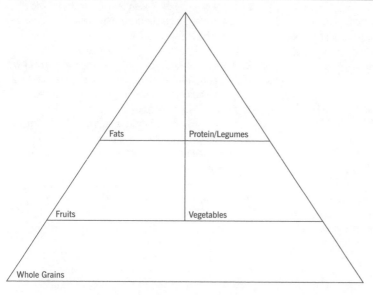

Fats
Protein/Legumes
Fruits
Vegetables
Whole Grains

Sunday

Breakfast

2 slices Fat-Free Banana Bread, 1 c. soy milk

Cal.: 410; Fat: 5.5 g; Protein: 12.4 g; Sodium: 323 mg; Fiber: 6.4 g; Carbs.: 79 g; Sugar: 33 g; Zinc: 0.4 mg; Calcium: 99.2 mg; Iron: 3.6 mg; Vit. D: 3 mcg; Vit. B$_{12}$: 0.41 mcg

Lunch

Hummus wrap with ½ c. spinach, ¼ c. tomatoes, 1 oz. olives, and ½ c. sprouts in a flour tortilla, 3 oz. baby carrots

Cal.: 265.8; Fat: 9 g; Protein: 8.63 g; Sodium: 755.2 mg; Fiber: 6.03 g; Carbs.: 40.25 g; Sugar: 7.05 g; Zinc: 0.55 mg; Calcium: 162.83 mg; Iron: 2.78 mg; Vit. D: 0 mcg; Vit. B$_{12}$: 0 mcg

Snack

3 oz. Spicy Roasted Chickpeas

Cal.: 116; Fat: 2.8 g; Protein: 4.2 g; Sodium: 371 mg; Fiber: 3.4 g; Carbs.: 19 g; Sugar: 0 g; Zinc: 0.83 mg; Calcium: 27 mg; Iron: 0.88 mg; Vit. D: 0 mcg; Vit. B$_{12}$: 0 mcg

Dinner

8 oz. White Spinach Lasagna, 1 c. steamed broccoli with 16 g nutritional yeast, 1 c. orange juice

Cal.: 648; Fat: 23.1 g; Protein: 35.3 g; Sodium: 796 mg; Fiber: 12.9 g; Carbs.: 87.1 g; Sugar: 26.5 g; Zinc: 6 mg; Calcium: 859 mg; Iron: 7.2 mg; Vit. D: 2.25 mcg; Vit. B$_{12}$: 8.63 mcg

Fat-Free Banana Bread

Yields 1 loaf

4 ripe bananas	1 t. baking powder
⅓ c. soy milk	½ t. baking soda
⅔ c. sugar	½ t. salt
1 t. vanilla	¾ t. cinnamon
2 c. all-purpose flour	

1. Preheat oven to 350°F. Lightly grease a loaf pan.
2. Mix together bananas, soy milk, sugar, and vanilla until smooth and creamy.
3. In a separate bowl, combine flour, baking powder, baking soda, and salt.
4. Combine the flour and banana mixtures until smooth.
5. Spread batter in loaf pan and sprinkle the top with cinnamon. Bake for about 55 minutes.

Spicy Roasted Chickpeas

Serves 5

1 (14-oz.) can chickpeas, drained and rinsed	½ t. chili powder
	¼ t. salt
2 t. olive oil	¼ t. cayenne pepper

1. Preheat oven to 350°F. Toss chickpeas with the oil to coat well. Add remaining ingredients and toss again.
2. Transfer chickpeas to a baking sheet and bake in the oven for 35–40 minutes, or until crunchy.

White Spinach Lasagna

Serves 4

½ onion, diced	2 c. soy milk
4 cloves garlic, minced	1 T. miso
2 T. olive oil	2 T. soy sauce
1 (10-oz.) box frozen spinach, thawed and pressed	2 T. lemon juice
	3 T. nutritional yeast
½ t. salt	2 t. onion powder
1 block firm tofu, crumbled	1 (12-oz.) package lasagna noodles
¾ c. cashew butter	

1. Sauté onion and garlic in olive oil until soft, add spinach and salt, stir to combine well. Cook until spinach is heated through. Add crumbled tofu and mix well. Allow to cool completely.
2. In a small saucepan over low heat, combine the cashew butter, soy milk, miso, soy sauce, lemon juice, nutritional yeast, and onion powder until smooth and creamy.
3. Prepare lasagna noodles according to package instructions, and pre-heat oven to 350°F.
4. In a lightly greased lasagna pan, layer cashew sauce, then noodles, then spinach, and repeat until all ingredients are used up. The top layer should be spinach and then sauce.
5. Bake for 40 minutes. Allow to cool for at least 10 minutes before serving, to allow lasagna to set.

Glasses of Water Consumed: _____

Thoughts About Today: _____

_____

_____

What I Ate Today

Time	Food Item	Amount	Calories	Fat	Carbs	Fiber	Protein
TOTAL							

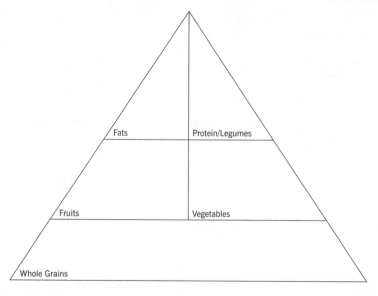

Fats

Protein/Legumes

Fruits

Vegetables

Whole Grains

WEEK 6 IN REVIEW

I feel: _____
_____
_____
_____

My greatest food discovery this week was: _____
_____
_____
_____

This week's biggest vegan challenge was: _____
_____
_____
_____

New food I'd like to try: _____
_____
_____
_____

When I look back at this week, I most want to remember: _____
_____
_____
_____

Nutrition Totals

	Calories	Fat	Carbs	Fiber	Protein
Goal					
Actual					

WEEK 7

You've learned quite a bit about preparing nutritious whole foods, have been eating a wide variety of fruits, vegetables, and healthy whole grains, and any cravings you have are beginning to subside. If not, you know plenty about meat and dairy substitutes and know how to satisfy a craving without giving up your fabulous new vegan diet.

Now that you've had plenty of time to ease into eating vegan, try adapting things a bit more to your personal tastes. Notice what works best for you, and begin listening to your own body and venturing out a bit more in the grocery store aisles. Try a few more store-bought substitutes, and, just for fun, see if you can find a vegetable or two you still haven't tried.

You know by now what foods are vegan, and which aren't, and you're used to eating well-balanced meals. Now that you're settled into your vegan ways, you're not likely to slip up, but you might find yourself getting bored, or just not caring. Now's the time to buy a new vegan cookbook to get inspired, subscribe to a few new e-newsletters, or just spend some extra time browsing online vegan forums or sites.

Let's keep a good thing going this week! You've made it this far—you can make it for life!

Monday

Breakfast

1 slice Fat-Free Banana Bread (see recipe in Week 6, Sun.), 1 small apple, 1 c. orange juice

Cal.: 347.5; Fat: 0.8 g; Protein: 5.1 g; Sodium: 148.5 mg; Fiber: 5.8 g; Carbs.: 81.6 g; Sugar: 53.5 g; Zinc: 0.3 mg; Calcium: 368.5 mg; Iron: 1.3 mg; Vit. D: 2.25 mcg; Vit. B_{12}: 0.47 mcg

Lunch

8 oz. leftover White Spinach Lasagna (see recipe in Week 6, Sun.), 1 small baked potato with 16 g nutritional yeast

Cal.: 617; Fat: 22.7 g; Protein: 33.5 g; Sodium: 796 mg; Fiber: 11.3 g; Carbs.: 80.2 g; Sugar: 4.2 g; Zinc: 5.9 mg; Calcium: 473.7 mg; Iron: 7.8 mg; Vit. D: 0 mcg; Vit. B_{12}: 8.63 mcg

Snack

Mixed veggies (½ cucumber, 2 oz. baby carrots, ½ c. broccoli) with 2 T. hummus

Cal.: 116.92; Fat: 3.32 g; Protein: 5.38 g; Sodium: 189.5 mg; Fiber: 6.52 g; Carbs.: 19.37 g; Sugar: 6.12 g; Zinc: 1.27 mg; Calcium: 81.63 mg; Iron: 2.18 mg; Vit. D: 0 mcg; Vit. B_{12}: 0 mcg

Dinner

1 c. Pineapple Glazed Tofu, 1 c. rice noodles

Cal.: 603; Fat: 18.4 g; Protein: 18.6 g; Sodium: 689.4 mg; Fiber: 4.4 g; Carbs.: 92.8 g; Sugar: 33 g; Zinc: 2.4 mg; Calcium: 716 mg; Iron: 3.5 mg; Vit. D: 0 mcg; Vit. B_{12}: 0 mcg

Pineapple Glazed Tofu

If you like orange chicken or sweet-and-sour dishes, try this saucy-sweet Pineapple Glazed Tofu, excellent for kids. Toss with some noodles, or add some diced veggies to make it an entrée. **Serves 3**

½ c. pineapple preserves
2 T. balsamic vinegar
2 T. soy sauce
⅔ c. pineapple juice
1 block firm or extra-firm tofu, cubed

3 T. flour
2 T. oil
1 t. cornstarch

1. Whisk together the pineapple preserves, vinegar, soy sauce, and pineapple juice.
2. Coat tofu in flour, then sauté in oil for a few minutes, just until lightly golden. Reduce heat to medium low and add pineapple sauce, stirring well to combine and coat tofu.
3. Heat for 3–4 minutes, stirring frequently, then add cornstarch, whisking to combine and avoid lumps. Heat for a few more minutes, stirring, until sauce has thickened.

Raising Healthy Vegan Kids Just like adults, vegan children have several health advantages when eating a plant-based diet. Even the American Dietetic Association agrees: "Well-planned vegan and other types of vegetarian diets are appropriate for all stages of the life cycle, including during pregnancy, lactation, infancy, childhood, and adolescence."

Date ____ / ____ / ____

Glasses of Water Consumed: _____

Thoughts About Today: _____

_____

_____

What I Ate Today

Time	Food Item	Amount	Calories	Fat	Carbs	Fiber	Protein
TOTAL							

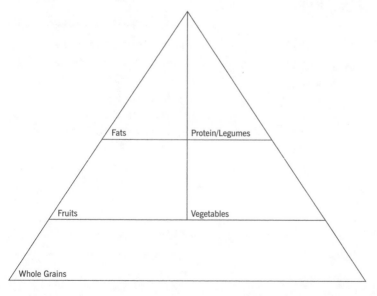

Tuesday

Breakfast

1 c. instant Cream of Wheat with 1 small banana, 1 c. soy hot chocolate

Cal.: 221.4; Fat: 2.9 g; Protein: 11.5 g; Sodium: 460 mg; Fiber: 5 g; Carbs.: 74.6 g; Sugar: 27.6 g; Zinc: 1.2 mg; Calcium: 459.1 mg; Iron: 13.38 mg; Vit. D: 2.7 mcg; Vit. B$_{12}$: 3 mcg

Lunch

1¾ c. Greek Salad with Tofu (see recipe in Week 2, Mon.) with 1 c. romaine lettuce, 1 c. pineapple, 1 c. applesauce

Cal.: 523.5; Fat: 26.4 g; Protein: 17.3 g; Sodium: 515.6 mg; Fiber: 9.6 g; Carbs.: 67.1 g; Sugar: 46.9 g; Zinc: 1.9 mg; Calcium: 624.3 mg; Iron: 4.1 mg; Vit. D: 0 mcg; Vit. B$_{12}$: 0 mcg

Snack

1 slice Fat-Free Banana Bread (see recipe in Week 6, Sun.), 1 oz. cashews

Cal.: 315; Fat: 12.8 g; Protein: 7.8 g; Sodium: 150.4 mg; Fiber: 3.1 g; Carbs.: 46.2 g; Sugar: 17.7 g; Zinc: 1.8 mg; Calcium: 20 mg; Iron: 3 mg; Vit. D: 0 mcg; Vit. B$_{12}$: 0.06 mcg

Dinner

6 oz. Massaman Curried Seitan, 1 c. brown rice

Cal.: 474; Fat: 20.3 g; Protein: 14.5 g; Sodium: 399.7 mg; Fiber: 3.5 g; Carbs.: 61.7 g; Sugar: 1.7 g; Zinc: 1.8 mg; Calcium: 59.5 mg; Iron: 3 mg; Vit. D: 0 mcg; Vit. B$_{12}$: 0 mcg

Massaman Curried Seitan

With Indian influences and popular among Muslim communities in Southern Thailand, massaman curry is a truly global dish. This version is simplified, but it still has a distinct kick. Diced tomatoes, baby corn, or green peas would go well in this recipe if you want to add veggies. **Serves 6**

1 T. Chinese Five-Spice powder	2 potatoes, chopped
½ t. fresh ginger, grated	1½ c. seitan, chopped small
½ t. turmeric	¼ t. cinnamon
¼ t. cayenne pepper, or to taste	2 whole cloves
1 T. oil	1 t. salt
1½ c. coconut milk	1 T. peanut butter
1 c. vegetable broth	2 t. brown sugar
	⅓ c. peanuts or cashews (optional)

1. In a large skillet or stockpot, heat five-spice powder, ginger, turmeric, and cayenne pepper in oil for just one minute, stirring constantly, until fragrant.
2. Reduce heat to medium low and add coconut milk and vegetable broth, stirring to combine. Add potatoes, seitan, cinnamon, cloves, and salt, cover, and cook for 15–20 minutes, stirring occasionally.
3. Uncover, add peanut butter, sugar, and peanuts or cashews, and heat for 1 more minute. Serve over rice.
4. If you prefer a thicker curry, dissolve 1 T. cornstarch in 3 T. water and add to curry, simmering for 2–3 minutes, until thick.

No More Boring Green Salads!

Stock up on vegan salad dressings (or make a few of your own) so you'll always be ready. Try a Mexican-themed green salad with crumbled tortilla chips, salsa, and avocado. Add corn kernels and black beans for a Tex-Mex feel, and season with chili powder. Go Greek with olives, red onions, fresh oregano, and artichoke hearts. Try a sweet treat salad with diced apples or tangerine slices, candied walnuts, and dried cranberries.

Glasses of Water Consumed: _____

Thoughts About Today: _____

_____

_____

What I Ate Today

Time	Food Item	Amount	Calories	Fat	Carbs	Fiber	Protein
TOTAL							

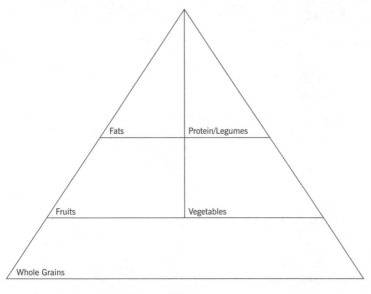

Fats

Protein/Legumes

Fruits

Vegetables

Whole Grains

Wednesday

Breakfast

1 English muffin with 1 vegan sausage patty, 1 (1-oz.) slice vegan cheese, 1 c. soy milk

Cal.: 427.5; Fat: 10.9 g; Protein: 23.8 g; Sodium: 658.5 mg; Fiber: 8.1 g; Carbs.: 61 g; Sugar: 19.3 g; Zinc: 0.8 mg; Calcium: 393.9 mg; Iron: 5.44 mg; Vit. D: 3 mcg; Vit. B$_{12}$: 2.46 mcg

Lunch

Rice salad with 1 c. leftover brown rice, 1 c. mixed veggies, and 2 T. Goddess Dressing (see recipe in Week 1, Mon.), 1 c. strawberries, 1 c. tomato juice

Cal.: 501.44; Fat: 16.94 g; Protein: 15.86 g; Sodium: 318.1 mg; Fiber: 18.11 g; Carbs.: 82.14 g; Sugar: 28.95 g; Zinc: 3.72 mg; Calcium: 262.21 mg; Iron: 6.78 mg; Vit. D: 0 mcg; Vit. B$_{12}$: 0 mcg

Snack

1 pita with 2 T. hummus

Cal.: 215; Fat: 3.5 g; Protein: 7.9 g; Sodium: 435.6 mg; Fiber: 3.1 g; Carbs.: 37.6 g; Sugar: 0.8 g; Zinc: 1.1 mg; Calcium: 63 mg; Iron: 2.4 mg; Vit. D: 0 mcg; Vit. B$_{12}$: 0 mcg

Dinner

½ Creamed Spinach and Mushrooms, 1 c. quinoa, 1 slice whole grain bread, toasted

Cal.: 402; Fat: 13.6 g; Protein: 14.6 g; Sodium: 159 mg; Fiber: 7.76 g; Carbs.: 55.5 g; Sugar: 2.34 g; Zinc: 2.94 mg; Calcium: 153.1 mg; Iron: 4.8 mg; Vit. D: 0 mcg; Vit. B$_{12}$: 0.62 mcg

Creamed Spinach and Mushrooms

The combination of greens and nutritional yeast is simply delicious and provides an excellent jolt of nutrients that vegans need. Don't forget that spinach will shrink when cooked, so use lots! **Serves 4**

½ onion, diced	1 c. soy milk
2 cloves garlic, minced	1 T. vegan margarine
1½ c. sliced mushrooms	¼ t. nutmeg (optional)
2 T. olive oil	2 T. nutritional yeast (optional)
1 T. flour	
2 bunches fresh spinach, trimmed	Salt and pepper, to taste

1. Sauté onion, garlic, and mushrooms in olive oil for 3–4 minutes. Add flour and heat, stirring constantly, for 1 minute.
2. Reduce heat to medium low and add spinach and soy milk. Cook uncovered for 8–10 minutes until spinach is soft and liquid has reduced.
3. Stir in remaining ingredients and season with salt and pepper to taste.

Wednesday

Glasses of Water Consumed: _____

Thoughts About Today: _____

_____

_____

What I Ate Today

Time	Food Item	Amount	Calories	Fat	Carbs	Fiber	Protein
TOTAL							

Fats

Protein/Legumes

Fruits

Vegetables

Whole Grains

Bored of Hummus? Spice it up by stirring in a few minced roasted red peppers, marinated garlic, sun-dried tomatoes, Indian seasonings, minced chipotles or jalapeños, or a sprinkle of fresh herbs—just about any kind will do.

Thursday

Breakfast

1½ c. Tropical Breakfast Couscous (see recipe in Week 2, Fri.), 1 banana, 1 c. soy milk

Cal.: 616.9; Fat: 29.8 g; Protein: 15.1 g; Sodium: 51 mg; Fiber: 5.6 g; Carbs.: 79.1 g; Sugar: 35.4 g; Zinc: 2.2 mg; Calcium: 123.1 mg; Iron: 3.1 mg; Vit. D: 3 mcg; Vit. B$_{12}$: 0.36 mcg

Lunch

Sandwich with 1 oz. Sun-Dried Tomato Pesto (see recipe in Week 2, Mon.), 1 oz. avocado, ¼ tomato, and 1 c. sprouts on 2 slices whole grain bread

Cal.: 391.93; Fat: 14.65 g; Protein: 14.48 g; Sodium: 602.55 mg; Fiber: 10.78 g; Carbs.: 55.3 g; Sugar: 19.8 g; Zinc: 1.25 mg; Calcium: 87.78 mg; Iron: 2.98 mg; Vit. D: 0 mcg; Vit. B$_{12}$: 0 mcg

Snack

1 oz. dried apricots, 2 oz. cashews

Cal.: 377.5; Fat: 24.7 g; Protein: 11.1 g; Sodium: 9.6 mg; Fiber: 3.8 g; Carbs.: 35.9 g; Sugar: 18.4 g; Zinc: 3.3 mg; Calcium: 36.2 mg; Iron: 4.5 mg; Vit. D: 0 mcg; Vit. B$_{12}$: 0 mcg

Dinner

1½ c. White Bean and Orzo Minestrone Soup

Cal.: 358.5; Fat: 6.75 g; Protein: 12.9 g; Sodium: 52.5 mg; Fiber: 10.35 g; Carbs.: 63 g; Sugar: 4.2 g; Zinc: 1.23 mg; Calcium: 1115.5 mg; Iron: 5.1 mg; Vit. D: 0 mcg; Vit. B$_{12}$: 0 mcg

White Bean and Orzo Minestrone Soup

Italian minestrone is a simple and universally loved soup. This version uses tiny orzo pasta, cannellini beans, and plenty of veggies. **Serves 6**

3 cloves garlic, minced
1 onion, chopped
2 ribs celery, chopped
2 T. olive oil
5 c. vegetable broth
1 carrot, diced
1 c. green beans, chopped
2 small potatoes, chopped small

2 tomatoes, chopped
1 (15-oz.) can cannellini beans, drained
1 t. basil
½ t. oregano
¾ c. orzo
Salt and pepper to taste

1. In a large soup pot, heat garlic, onion, and celery in olive oil until just soft, about 3–4 minutes.
2. Add vegetable broth, carrot, green beans, potatoes, tomatoes, beans, basil, and oregano, and bring to a simmer. Cover, and cook on medium low heat for 20–25 minutes.
3. Add orzo and heat another 10 minutes, just until orzo is cooked. Season well with salt and pepper.

Date ____ / ____ / ____

Glasses of Water Consumed: _____

Thoughts About Today: _____

_____

_____

What I Ate Today

Time	Food Item	Amount	Calories	Fat	Carbs	Fiber	Protein
TOTAL							

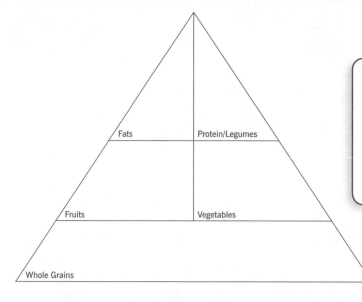

Sandwich Substitutes Vegetarian deli meat slices are hit-and-miss. Some are chewy and savory, while others taste like plastic in your mouth. Tofurky deli slices are one popular brand, but try a couple of different ones to see what you like.

Friday

Breakfast

½ c. baked beans on 2 slices whole grain toast, 1 small apple

Cal.: 266.6; Fat: 1.9 g; Protein: 9.9 g; Sodium: 591.5 mg; Fiber: 11.5 g; Carbs.: 55.9 g; Sugar: 26.2 g; Zinc: 2.6 mg; Calcium: 75.5 mg; Iron: 3.6 mg; Vit. D: 0 mcg; Vit. B$_{12}$: 0 mcg

Lunch

1½ c. leftover White Bean and Orzo Minestrone Soup (see recipe in Week 7, Thurs.)

Cal.: 358.5; Fat: 6.75 g; Protein: 12.9 g; Sodium: 52.5 mg; Fiber: 10.35 g; Carbs.: 63 g; Sugar: 4.2 g; Zinc: 1.23 mg; Calcium: 1115.5 mg; Iron: 5.1 mg; Vit. D: 0 mcg; Vit. B$_{12}$: 0 mcg

Snack

1 c. yogurt with ⅓ c. granola, 1 oz. almonds

Cal.: 495; Fat: 26.3 g; Protein: 16.1 g; Sodium: 91.4 mg; Fiber: 7.6 g; Carbs.: 57.3 g; Sugar: 27.8 g; Zinc: 2.1 mg; Calcium: 118.6 mg; Iron: 2.4 mg; Vit. D: 0 mcg; Vit. B$_{12}$: 0 mcg

Dinner

6 oz. Easy Pad Thai Noodles

Cal.: 333; Fat: 19 g; Protein: 13 g; Sodium: 998 mg; Fiber: 3 g; Carbs.: 32 g; Sugar: 6.6 g; Zinc: 1.6 mg; Calcium: 419 mg; Iron: 2.3 mg; Vit. D: 0.79 mcg; Vit. B$_{12}$: 0 mcg

Easy Pad Thai Noodles

Volumes could be written about Thailand's national dish. It's sweet, sour, spicy, and salty all at once, and filled with as much texture and flavor as the streets of Bangkok themselves. **Serves 6**

1 lb thin rice noodles

Hot water for soaking

¼ c. tahini

¼ c. ketchup

¼ c. soy sauce

2 T. white, rice, or cider vinegar

3 T. lime juice

2 T. sugar

¾ t. crushed red pepper flakes or cayenne pepper

1 block firm or extra-firm tofu, diced small

3 cloves garlic

¼ c. vegetable or safflower oil

4 scallions, chopped

½ t. salt

Optional toppings: bean sprouts, crushed toasted peanuts, extra scallions, sliced lime

1. Cover the noodles in hot water and set aside to soak until soft, about 5 minutes.
2. Whisk together the tahini, ketchup, soy sauce, vinegar, lime juice, sugar, and red pepper flakes.
3. In a large skillet, fry the tofu and garlic in oil until tofu is lightly golden brown. Add noodles, stirring to combine well, and fry for 2–3 minutes.
4. Reduce heat to medium and add tahini and ketchup sauce mixture, stirring well to combine. Allow to cook for 3–4 minutes, until well combined and heated through. Add green onions and salt and heat 1 more minute, stirring well.
5. Serve with extra chopped scallions, bean sprouts, crushed peanuts, and a lime wedge or two.

Glasses of Water Consumed: _____

Thoughts About Today: _____

_____

_____

What I Ate Today

Time	Food Item	Amount	Calories	Fat	Carbs	Fiber	Protein
TOTAL							

Fats

Protein/Legumes

Fruits

Vegetables

Whole Grains

Know Your Noodles Noodles cook quicker than pasta, so they're great when you're super-hungry or in a hurry. Many grocery stores even stock shirataki noodles—a high-protein, low-carb noodle made from tofu that doesn't need to be cooked—perfect for hungry vegans to slurp! Check the refrigerator section for these.

Saturday

Breakfast

6 oz. Baked "Sausage" and Mushroom Frittata, 1 small banana

Cal.: 381.9; Fat: 20.3 g; Protein: 23.1 g; Sodium: 1182 mg; Fiber: 5.6 g; Carbs.: 32.9 g; Sugar: 12.77 g; Zinc: 2.4 mg; Calcium: 421.1 mg; Iron: 4.6 mg; Vit. D: 0 mcg; Vit. B$_{12}$: 0.06 mcg

Lunch

6 oz. leftover Easy Pad Thai Noodles (see recipe in Week 7, Fri.)

Cal.: 333; Fat: 19 g; Protein: 13 g; Sodium: 998 mg; Fiber: 3 g; Carbs.: 32 g; Sugar: 6.6 g; Zinc: 1.6 mg; Calcium: 419 mg; Iron: 2.3 mg; Vit. D: 0.79 mcg; Vit. B$_{12}$: 0 mcg

Snack

1 c. edamame, 2 oz. dried cranberries

Cal.: 275; Fat: 8.5 g; Protein: 16.9 g; Sodium: 10.1 mg; Fiber: 9.7 g; Carbs.: 38.9 g; Sugar: 21.6 g; Zinc: 2.1 mg; Calcium: 100.4 mg; Iron: 3.6 mg; Vit. D: 0 mcg; Vit. B$_{12}$: 0 mcg

Dinner

5 oz. Super-Quick Black Bean Soup, 1 c. roasted butternut squash

Cal.: 505; Fat: 2 g; Protein: 28.8 g; Sodium: 75.2 mg; Fiber: 19 g; Carbs.: 98.5 g; Sugar: 6.5 g; Zinc: 5.2 mg; Calcium: 236 mg; Iron: 7.6 mg; Vit. D: 0 mcg; Vit. B$_{12}$: 0 mcg

Baked "Sausage" and Mushroom Frittata

Baked tofu frittatas are an easy brunch or weekend breakfast. Once you've got the technique down, it's easy to adjust the ingredients to your liking. With tofu and mock meat, this one packs a super protein punch!

Serves 6

½ yellow onion, diced

3 gloves garlic, minced

½ c. sliced mushrooms

1 (12-oz.) package vegetarian sausage substitute or vegetarian "beef" crumbles

2 T. olive oil

¾ t. salt

¼ t. black pepper

1 block firm or extra-firm tofu

1 block silken tofu

1 T. soy sauce

2 T. nutritional yeast

¼ t. turmeric (optional)

1 tomato, sliced thin (optional)

1. Preheat oven to 325°F and lightly grease a glass pie pan.
2. Heat onion, garlic, mushrooms, and vegetarian sausage in olive oil in a large skillet for 3–4 minutes, until sausage is browned and mushrooms are soft. Season with salt and pepper and set aside.
3. Combine firm tofu, silken tofu, soy sauce, nutritional yeast, and turmeric in a blender, and process until mixed. Combine tofu with sausage mixture and spread into pan. Layer slices of tomato on top (optional).
4. Bake in oven for about 45 minutes, or until firm. Allow to cool for 5–10 minutes before serving, as frittata will set as it cools.

Super-Quick Black Bean Soup

Serves 6

2 (15-oz.) cans black beans, undrained

1 c. vegetable broth

⅔ c. salsa

½ t. garlic powder

1 T. chili powder

Dash salt

1 T. chopped fresh cilantro

1. Using a potato masher or a large fork, coarsely mash one can of beans.
2. In a medium saucepan, combine the mashed beans with the remaining whole beans, vegetable broth, salsa, garlic powder, chili powder, and salt. Simmer for a few minutes, just until well combined and heated through. Serve topped with fresh chopped cilantro.

Glasses of Water Consumed: _____

Thoughts About Today: _____

_____

_____

What I Ate Today

Time	Food Item	Amount	Calories	Fat	Carbs	Fiber	Protein
TOTAL							

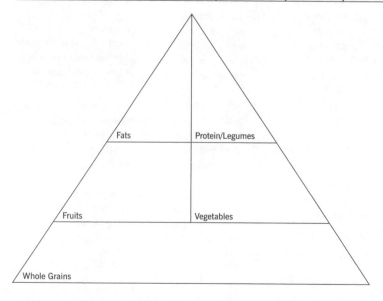

Sunday

Breakfast

1 Blueberry Muffin, mixed fruit salad with ¼ c. grapes, ½ tangerine, ½ diced apple, ½ banana, ¼ c. chopped cantaloupe, 1 c. soy milk

Cal.: 348; Fat: 5.94 g; Protein: 12.3 g; Sodium: 177 mg; Fiber: 9.4 g; Carbs.: 67 g; Sugar: 33.5 g; Zinc: 0.51 mg; Calcium: 151 mg; Iron: 2.4 mg; Vit. D: 3 mcg; Vit. B$_{12}$: 0.61 mcg

Lunch

5 oz. leftover Super-Quick Black Bean Soup (see recipe in Week 7, Sat.), ½ lb collard greens sautéed with ½ T. oil, 1 clove garlic, and 16 g nutritional yeast, 1 slice whole grain toast

Cal.: 677.1; Fat: 11.2 g; Protein: 44.5 g; Sodium: 520 mg; Fiber: 33.3 g; Carbs.: 108.9 g; Sugar: 6.32 g; Zinc: 8.68 mg; Calcium: 522.6 mg; Iron: 8.46 mg; Vit. D: 0 mcg; Vit. B$_{12}$: 7.8 mcg

Snack

9 oz. Fresh Basil Bruschetta

Cal.: 314; Fat: 8.9 g; Protein: 6.9 g; Sodium: 398 mg; Fiber: 3 g; Carbs.: 53 g; Sugar: 18 g; Zinc: 0.69 mg; Calcium: 65 mg; Iron: 2.1 mg; Vit. D: 0 mcg; Vit. B$_{12}$: 0 mcg

Dinner

10 oz. Sweet-and-Sour Tempeh, ½ c. brown rice or quinoa

Cal.: 491; Fat: 14.8 g; Protein: 17 g; Sodium: 580.8 mg; Fiber: 5.8 g; Carbs.: 72.8 g; Sugar: 15.7 g; Zinc: 2.19 mg; Calcium: 114.5 mg; Iron: 3.4 mg; Vit. D: 0 mcg; Vit. B$_{12}$: 0 mcg

Blueberry Muffins

Yields approx 1½ dozen muffins

2 c. whole wheat flour	1½ c. soy milk
1 c. all-purpose flour	½ c. applesauce
1¼ c. sugar	½ t. vanilla
1 T. baking powder	2 c. blueberries
1 t. salt	

1. Preheat oven to 400°F. In a large bowl, combine the flours, sugar, baking powder, and salt. Set aside.
2. Combine wet ingredients, and whisk until mixed.
3. Combine wet and dry ingredients. Stir until mixed. Fold in 1 c. blueberries. Fill lined muffin tins 2" full with batter. Top with 1 c. blueberries.
4. Bake for 20–25 minutes, or until lightly golden.

Fresh Basil Bruschetta

Serves 4

¾ c. balsamic vinegar	2 T. olive oil
1 T. sugar	¼ c. chopped fresh basil
2 large tomatoes, diced	Salt and pepper to taste
3 cloves garlic, minced	8–10 slices French bread

1. Whisk vinegar and sugar in saucepan. Boil, then simmer for 6-8 minutes to reduce. Remove from heat.
2. Combine tomatoes, garlic, olive oil, basil, salt, and pepper in bowl. Gently toss with balsamic sauce.
3. Spoon tomato and balsamic mixture over bread.

Sweet-and-Sour Tempeh

Serves 4

1 c. vegetable broth	1 T. cornstarch
2 T. soy sauce	2 T. olive oil
1 (8-oz.) pkg tempeh	1 green bell pepper, chopped
2 T. barbecue sauce	1 red bell pepper, chopped
½ t. ground ginger	1 yellow onion, chopped
2 T. maple syrup	1 (15-oz.) can pineapple chunks, reserve juice
⅓ c. rice vinegar	

1. Whisk broth and soy sauce. Bring to simmer in large skillet. Add tempeh and simmer for 10 minutes. Remove tempeh from pan. Reserve ½ c. broth mix.
2. In a small bowl, whisk the barbecue sauce, ginger, maple syrup, vinegar, cornstarch, and juice from pineapples until cornstarch is dissolved. Set aside.
3. Heat oil, tempeh, peppers, and onion in skillet. Sauté for 1 minute. Add sauce and bring to simmer.
4. Allow to cook until sauce thickens, about 6–8 minutes. Reduce heat and stir in pineapples.

Date ____ / ____ / ____

Sunday

Glasses of Water Consumed: _____

Thoughts About Today: _____

_____

_____

What I Ate Today

Time	Food Item	Amount	Calories	Fat	Carbs	Fiber	Protein
TOTAL							

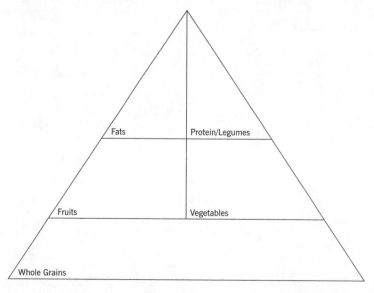

Fats

Protein/Legumes

Fruits

Vegetables

Whole Grains

WEEK 7 IN REVIEW

I feel: _____
_____
_____
_____

My greatest food discovery this week was: _____
_____
_____
_____

This week's biggest vegan challenge was: _____
_____
_____
_____

New food I'd like to try: _____
_____
_____
_____

When I look back at this week, I most want to remember: ____
_____
_____
_____

Nutrition Totals

	Calories	Fat	Carbs	Fiber	Protein
Goal					
Actual					

WEEK 8

You've been vegan almost two months now, can you believe it? You're two-thirds of the way through this planner, and hopefully well on the way to achieving your goals. How does it feel? Sometimes, our daily lives are so hectic and busy that we barely have a moment to stop and relax, much less to really take time out to think. This week, set aside an hour or two to take a mental relaxation break. Find a quiet spot or go for a meditative walk, whether it's at a city park, the beach, or a mountain trail. Turn off your cell phone and just be. Let your mind process the journey that you've undertaken, and appreciate just how far you've come and changed as a person. Reflect on how your experiences over the past eight weeks have changed you, and what you hope to achieve over the next few weeks to come. Are you happy as a vegan? Was it easier or harder than you thought? Has it been worth it so far? Is it more or less fulfilling than you thought it would be? What will be the next step for you?

If this isn't something you normally do, you'll be surprised just how nourishing an hour or two of fresh air, nature, and mental solitude can be. Don't forget to pack a healthy snack!

Monday

Breakfast

2 Blueberry Muffins (see recipe in Week 7, Sun.), 1 small banana, 1 c. soy milk

Cal.: 383.9; Fat: 6.24 g; Protein: 14.7 g; Sodium: 306 mg; Fiber: 9 g; Carbs.: 72.1 g; Sugar: 22.4 g; Zinc: 1.22 mg; Calcium: 159.4 mg; Iron: 3.7 mg; Vit. D: 3 mcg; Vit. B$_{12}$: 0.86 mcg

Lunch

1 c. store-bought vegetarian chili (approximately 250 calories), 1 c. steamed broccoli with 16 g nutritional yeast

Record nutritional values for your choice of vegetarian chili in today's journal. The nutritional values below are for steamed broccoli and nutritional yeast only.

Cal.: 94; Fat: 1.1 g; Protein: 11.3 g; Sodium: 5 mg; Fiber: 8.6 g; Carbs.: 15.1 g; Sugar: 2.9 g; Zinc: 3.6 mg; Calcium: 556 mg; Iron: 1.6 mg; Vit. D: 0 mcg; Vit. B$_{12}$: 7.8 mcg

Snack

Mixed veggies (½ cucumber, 2 oz. baby carrots, ½ c. broccoli) with 2 T. hummus

Cal.: 116.92; Fat: 3.32 g; Protein: 5.38 g; Sodium: 189.5 mg; Fiber: 6.52 g; Carbs.: 19.37 g; Sugar: 6.12 g; Zinc: 1.27 mg; Calcium: 81.63 mg; Iron: 2.18 mg; Vit. D: 0 mcg; Vit. B$_{12}$: 0 mcg

Dinner

1 c. Vietnamese Noodle Salad, 1 c. steamed spinach, 1 c. orange juice

Cal.: 358.4; Fat: 1.5 g; Protein: 10.3 g; Sodium: 853 mg; Fiber: 6.8 g; Carbs.: 80.7 g; Sugar: 24.3 g; Zinc: mg; Calcium: 1.52 mg; Iron: 640 mg; Vit. D: 10.65 mcg; Vit. B$_{12}$: 0.41 mcg

Vietnamese Noodle Salad

Serves 2

1 vegetarian chicken cutlets

4 oz. bean thread noodles, softened in hot water for 20 minutes

½ c. thinly sliced scallions

½ c. fresh cilantro

1–2 T. crushed red pepper flakes

2 T. lime juice

2 T. soy sauce

1 T. pickled garlic, chopped

Sugar to taste

1. Grill the vegetarian chicken cutlet for a few minutes on each side (or according to package instructions), until well marked, then chop into thin strips.
2. Drain the soaked and softened noodles. Combine the noodles, chicken strips, scallions, cilantro, and crushed red pepper into a serving bowl.
3. Mix together the lime juice, soy sauce, pickled garlic, and sugar, and toss with the salad ingredients.

The Perfect Green If you think spinach is too slimy and kale is too bitter, have you tried Swiss chard? It's quicker-cooking than collards, but with a milder flavor than kale or mustard greens. Try it steamed with a bit of garlic, olive oil, and lemon juice, or smothered in nutritional yeast or vegan Parmesan.

Glasses of Water Consumed: _____

Thoughts About Today: _____

_____

_____

What I Ate Today

Time	Food Item	Amount	Calories	Fat	Carbs	Fiber	Protein
TOTAL							

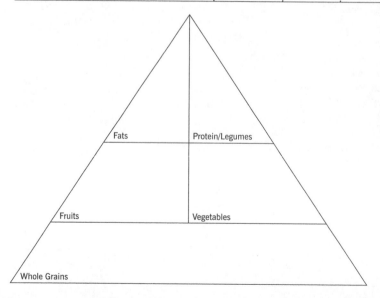

Fats

Protein/Legumes

Fruits

Vegetables

Whole Grains

Tuesday

Breakfast

1 c. whole grain cereal with ½ c. soy milk

Cal.: 178.33; Fat: 2.92 g; Protein: 6.17 g; Sodium: 267.83 mg; Fiber: 4.6 g; Carbs.: 33.43 g; Sugar: 7.17 g; Zinc: 20 mg; Calcium: 1373.33 mg; Iron: 247.7 mg; Vit. D: 54.7 mcg; Vit. B_{12}: 8.18 mcg

Lunch

1 c. store-bought vegan baked beans, 1 c. pineapple, 1 slice whole grain toast

Record nutritional values for your choice of vegan baked beans in today's journal. The nutritional values below are for pineapple and toast only.

Cal.: 220.7; Fat: 2.4 g; Protein: 7.9 g; Sodium: 221.7 mg; Fiber: 6.1 g; Carbs.: 44.2 g; Sugar: 19.7 g; Zinc: 1 mg; Calcium: 74.7 mg; Iron: 1.9 mg; Vit. D: 0 mcg; Vit. B_{12}: 0 mcg

Snack

200 calories of pretzels, mixed fruit salad with ½ apple, ½ banana, ½ c. strawberries, and ½ c. pineapple

Record nutritional values for your choice of pretzels in today's journal. The nutritional values below are for mixed fruit salad only.

Cal.: 149.25; Fat: 0.65 g; Protein: 1.7 g; Sodium: 2.85 mg; Fiber: 5.75 g; Carbs.: 38.5 g; Sugar: 25.8 g; Zinc: 0.35 mg; Calcium: 29.9 mg; Iron: 0.8 mg; Vit. D: 0 mcg; Vit. B_{12}: 0 mcg

Dinner

17 oz. Spaghetti with Italian "Meatballs"

Cal.: 573; Fat: 17 g; Protein: 15 g; Sodium: 1884 mg; Fiber: 14 g; Carbs.: 91 g; Sugar: 33 g; Zinc: 2 mg; Calcium: 29 mg; Iron: 2 mg; Vit. D: 0 mcg; Vit. B_{12}: 0 mcg

Spaghetti with Italian "Meatballs"

These little TVP nuggets are so chewy and addicting, you just might want to make a double batch. If you can't find beef-flavored bouillon, just use what you've got. Don't be tempted to add extra water to the TVP, as it needs to be a little dry for this recipe. **Serves 4**

½ vegetarian beef-flavored bouillon cube (optional)	1 t. parsley
	½ t. sage
⅔ c. hot water	½ t. salt
⅔ c. TVP	½ c. bread crumbs
Egg replacer for 2 eggs	⅔–¾ c. flour
½ onion, minced	Oil for pan-frying
2 T. ketchup or barbecue sauce	1 12 oz. package spaghetti noodles, cooked
½ t. garlic powder	3 c. prepared spaghetti sauce
1 t. basil	

1. Dissolve bouillon cube in hot water, and pour over TVP to reconstitute. Allow to sit for 6–7 minutes. Gently press to remove any excess moisture.
2. In a large bowl, combine the TVP, egg replacer, onion, ketchup or barbecue sauce, and seasonings until well mixed.
3. Add bread crumbs and combine well, then add flour, a few tablespoons at a time, mixing well to combine until mixture is sticky and thick. You may need a little more or less than ⅔ cup.
4. Using lightly floured hands, shape into balls 1½–2 inches thick.
5. Pan-fry "meatballs" in a bit of oil over medium heat, rolling them around in the pan to maintain the shape, until golden brown on all sides.
6. Reduce heat to medium low and add spaghetti sauce, heating thoroughly. Serve over cooked spaghetti noodles.

Glasses of Water Consumed: _____

Thoughts About Today: _____

_____

_____

What I Ate Today

Time	Food Item	Amount	Calories	Fat	Carbs	Fiber	Protein
TOTAL							

Fats

Protein/Legumes

Fruits

Vegetables

Whole Grains

Human Rights, Animal Rights Many social-justice activists, including notable heroes Coretta Scott King and César Chévez, have rejected animal exploitation as a logical extension of their belief in equality. In the words of Albert Einstein, they have "widened the circle of compassion" to include all victims of oppression and injustice—animals and humans alike.

Wednesday

Breakfast

2 T. vegan cream cheese, 1 T. sugar-free jam on 2 slices whole grain toast, 1 c. tomato juice

Cal.: 279.2; Fat: 10.3 g; Protein: 10.8 g; Sodium: 359.3 mg; Fiber: 6.8 g; Carbs.: 40.9 g; Sugar: 13 g; Zinc: 1.2 mg; Calcium: 97.5 mg; Iron: 2.76 mg; Vit. D: 0 mcg; Vit. B$_{12}$: 0 mcg

Lunch

1 baked potato with ½ c. black beans, ¼ c. salsa, 1 oz. vegan cheese, 1 c. orange juice

Cal.: 231.4; Fat: 0.9 g; Protein: 7.5 g; Sodium: 365 mg; Fiber: 4 g; Carbs.: 80.6 g; Sugar: 34.6 g; Zinc: 0.6 mg; Calcium: 509.1 mg; Iron: 12.3 mg; Vit. D: 0 mcg; Vit. B$_{12}$: 0.41 mcg

Snack

200 calories of whole grain crackers with 2 T. almond butter

Record nutritional values for your choice of whole grain cracker in today's journal. The nutritional values below are for almond butter only.

Cal.: 101; Fat: 9.5 g; Protein: 2.4 g; Sodium: 1.8 mg; Fiber: 0.6 g; Carbs.: 3.4 g; Sugar: 0 g; Zinc: 0.5 mg; Calcium: 43.2 mg; Iron: 0.6 mg; Vit. D: 0 mcg; Vit. B$_{12}$: 0 mcg

Dinner

6¼ oz. Indian Tofu Palak with ½ c. quinoa and 16 g nutritional yeast

Cal.: 502; Fat: 19.1 g; Protein: 34.1 g; Sodium: 685 mg; Fiber: 12.1 g; Carbs.: 56.4 g; Sugar: 1.43 g; Zinc: 7.4 mg; Calcium: 677.5 mg; Iron: 9.1 0mg; Vit. D: 0 mcg; Vit. B$_{12}$: 7.8 mcg

Indian Tofu Palak

Palak paneer is a popular Indian dish of creamed spinach and soft cheese. This version uses tofu for a similar dish. **Serves 4**

3 cloves garlic, minced	4 bunches fresh spinach
1 block firm or extra firm tofu, cut into small cubes	3 T. water
	1 T. curry powder
2 T. olive oil	2 t. cumin
2 T. nutritional yeast	½ t. salt
½ t. onion powder	½ c. plain soy yogurt

1. Heat garlic and tofu in olive oil over low heat and add nutritional yeast and onion powder, stirring to coat tofu. Heat for 2–3 minutes, until tofu is lightly browned.
2. Add spinach, water, curry powder, cumin, and salt, stirring well to combine. Once spinach starts to wilt, add soy yogurt and heat just until spinach is fully wilted and soft.

Indian Vegan Options In India, many vegetarians forswear eggs as well as onions and garlic for religious purposes, making Indian food an excellent choice for vegans. When eating at Indian restaurants, be sure to ask about *ghee*, or Indian butter, which is a traditional ingredient, but easily and frequently substituted with oil.

Glasses of Water Consumed: _____

Thoughts About Today: _____

_____

_____

What I Ate Today

Time	Food Item	Amount	Calories	Fat	Carbs	Fiber	Protein
TOTAL							

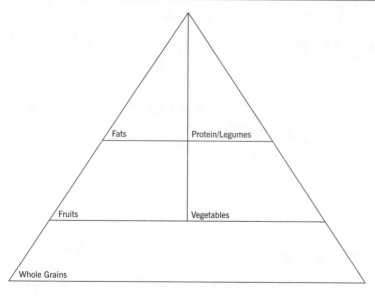

Thursday

Breakfast

½ c. oatmeal with 1 oz. almonds, 1 sliced banana, 1 c. soy milk

Cal.: 535.83; Fat: 19.4 g; Protein: 18 g; Sodium: 97.5 mg; Fiber: 7.4 g; Carbs.: 11 g; Sugar: 37.99 g; Zinc: 2.25 mg; Calcium: 387.93 mg; Iron: 3.34 mg; Vit. D: 2.7 mcg; Vit. B$_{12}$: 3 mcg

Lunch

6¼ oz. leftover Indian Tofu Palak (see recipe in Week 8, Wed.) with ½ c. quinoa

Cal.: 457; Fat: 18.6 g; Protein: 26.1 g; Sodium: 680 mg; Fiber: 8.1 g; Carbs.: 51.4 g; Sugar: 0.43 g; Zinc: 4.4 mg; Calcium: 677.5 mg; Iron: 8.4 mg; Vit. D: 0 mcg; Vit. B$_{12}$: 0 mcg

Snack

1 c. unsweetened applesauce, 1 oz. raisins

Cal.: 186.5; Fat: 0.3 g; Protein: 1.3 g; Sodium: 8 mg; Fiber: 3.7 g; Carbs.: 49.9 g; Sugar: 39.6 g; Zinc: 0.2 mg; Calcium: 23.9 mg; Iron: 1.1 mg; Vit. D: 0 mcg; Vit. B$_{12}$: 0 mcg

Dinner

6 oz. Sweet and Spicy Peanut Noodles, 1 c. steamed broccoli

Cal.: 531; Fat: 16.6 g; Protein: 21.3 g; Sodium: 1273 mg; Fiber: 6 g; Carbs.: 85.1 g; Sugar: 8.2 g; Zinc: 3 mg; Calcium: 105 mg; Iron: 4.1 mg; Vit. D: 0 mcg; Vit. B$_{12}$: 0 mcg

Sweet and Spicy Peanut Noodles

Like the call of the siren, these noodles entice you with their sweet pineapple flavor, then scorch your tongue with fiery chilies. Very sneaky, indeed. **Serves 4**

1 (12-oz.) package Asian-style noodles
⅓ c. peanut butter
2 T. soy sauce
⅔ c. pineapple juice
2 cloves garlic, minced

1 t. fresh ginger, grated
½ t. salt
1 T. olive oil
1 t. sesame oil
2–3 small chilies, minced
¾ c. diced pineapple

1. Prepare noodles according to package instructions and set aside.
2. In a small saucepan, stir together the peanut butter, soy sauce, pineapple juice, garlic, ginger, and salt over low heat, just until well combined.
3. Place the olive oil and sesame oil in a large skillet and fry minced chilies and pineapple for 2–3 minutes, stirring frequently, until pineapple is lightly browned. Add noodles and fry for another minute, stirring well.
4. Reduce heat to low and add peanut butter sauce mixture, stirring to combine well. Heat for 1 more minute, until well combined.

Stay Motivated, Stay Informed

Bored and online? Take a few minutes to learn something new without cracking a book. YouTube is full of vegan cooking demonstrations, lectures, interviews, and plenty of pure comedic gold. Just type the word *vegan* into YouTube, and you'll be entertained for hours.

Glasses of Water Consumed: _____

Thoughts About Today: _____

_____

_____

What I Ate Today

Time	Food Item	Amount	Calories	Fat	Carbs	Fiber	Protein
TOTAL							

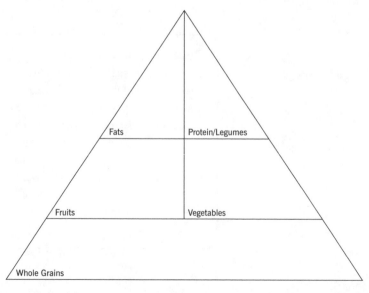

Friday

Breakfast

1 c. Cream of Wheat with 1 small banana, 1 c. soy hot chocolate

Cal.: 221.4; Fat: 2.9 g; Protein: 11.5 g; Sodium: 460 mg; Fiber: 5 g; Carbs.: 74.6 g; Sugar: 27.6 g; Zinc: 1.2 mg; Calcium: 459.1 mg; Iron: 13.38 mg; Vit. D: 2.7 mcg; Vit. B$_{12}$: 3 mcg

Lunch

6 oz. leftover Sweet and Spicy Peanut Noodles (see recipe in Week 8, Thurs.), 1 c. pineapple

Cal.: 564.5; Fat: 16.2 g; Protein: 18.9 g; Sodium: 1274.7 mg; Fiber: 3.7 g; Carbs.: 96.6 g; Sugar: 22.6 g; Zinc: 2.6 mg; Calcium: 70.5 mg; Iron: 3.7 mg; Vit. D: 0 mcg; Vit. B$_{12}$: 0 mcg

Snack

200 calories of whole grain chips with ½ c. salsa

Record nutritional values for your choice of whole grain chips and salsa in today's journal.

Dinner

½ c. Homemade Garlic and Herb Gnocchi with 1 oz. Sun-Dried Tomato Pesto (see recipe in Week 2, Mon.), side green salad with 2 c. romaine lettuce, 1 tomato, and 1 diced cucumber, 2 T. Goddess Dressing (see recipe in Week 1, Mon.)

Cal.: 546.2; Fat: 20.77 g; Protein: 16.8 g; Sodium: 1045.2 mg; Fiber: 9.12 g; Carbs.: 77.9 g; Sugar: 10.89 g; Zinc: 2.06 mg; Calcium: 178.5 mg; Iron: 7.22 mg; Vit. D: 0 mcg; Vit. B$_{12}$: 0 mcg

Homemade Garlic and Herb Gnocchi

Homemade gnocchi is well worth the effort if you have the time! **Serves 4**

2 large potatoes
¾ t. garlic powder
½ t. dried basil
½ t. dried parsley
¾ t. salt
1½ c. all-purpose flour
Water for boiling

1. Microwave or bake potatoes until done, about 50 minutes at 400°F. Allow to cool, then peel skins.
2. Using a fork, mash potatoes with garlic powder, basil, parsley, and salt until potatoes are completely smooth, with no lumps.
3. On a floured work surface, place half of the flour, and the potatoes on top. Use your hands to work the flour into the potatoes to form a dough. Only add as much flour as is needed to form a dough. Knead smooth.
4. Working in batches, roll out a rope of dough about 1 inch thick. Slice into 1-inch-long pieces, and gently roll against a fork to make grooves in the dough. This helps the sauce stick to the dough.
5. Cook gnocchi in boiling water for 2–3 minutes, until they rise to the surface. Serve immediately.

Baked Tortilla Chips Instead of a bag of chips, grab a bag of whole wheat tortillas at the store, and make your own tortilla chips! Slice the tortillas into strips or triangles, and arrange in a single layer on a baking sheet. Drizzle with olive oil for a crispier chip, and season with a bit of salt and garlic powder if you want, or just bake them plain. It'll take about 5–6 minutes on each side in a 300°F oven.

Glasses of Water Consumed: _____

Thoughts About Today: _____

_____

_____

What I Ate Today

Time	Food Item	Amount	Calories	Fat	Carbs	Fiber	Protein
TOTAL							

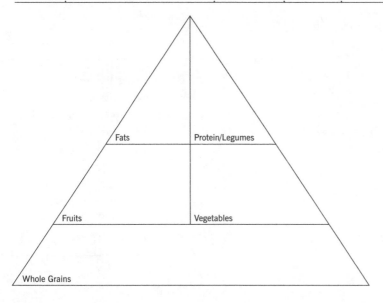

Fats

Protein/Legumes

Fruits

Vegetables

Whole Grains

Saturday

Breakfast

1 vegan sausage patty, 2 Quick and Easy Vegan Biscuits, 2 T. sugar-free jam

Cal.: 207; Fat: 7.4 g; Protein: 12.2 g; Sodium: 89 mg; Fiber: 1.56 g; Carbs.: 28 g; Sugar: 1 g; Zinc: 0.22 mg; Calcium: 71 mg; Iron: 2.54 mg; Vit. D: 0 mcg; Vit. B_{12}: 2.25 mcg

Lunch

Vegan grilled cheese sandwich, side green salad with 2 c. romaine lettuce, 1 tomato, and 1 diced cucumber, 2 T. Goddess Dressing (see recipe in Week 1, Mon.)

Cal.: 498.2; Fat: 18.8 g; Protein: 15.9 g; Sodium: 687.7 mg; Fiber: 13.52 g; Carbs.: 75.1 g; Sugar: 28.66 g; Zinc: 2.48 mg; Calcium: 605.6 mg; Iron: 4.92 mg; Vit. D: 0 mcg; Vit. B_{12}: 0 mcg

Snack

1 pita, mixed veggies (½ cucumber, 2 oz. baby carrots, ½ c. broccoli) with 2 T. hummus

Cal.: 306.92; Fat: 5.42 g; Protein: 12.08 g; Sodium: 568.3 mg; Fiber: 8.72 g; Carbs.: 54.87 g; Sugar: 6.92 g; Zinc: 2.07 mg; Calcium: 138.93 mg; Iron: 4.18 mg; Vit. D: 0 mcg; Vit. B_{12}: 0 mcg

Dinner

Store-bought vegetarian chicken nuggets (about 450 calories), vegan mashed potatoes, 8 spears steamed asparagus

Record nutritional values for vegetarian chicken nuggets in today's journal. The nutritional values below are for potatoes and asparagus only.

Cal.: 154.4; Fat: 0.4 g; Protein: 6.3 g; Sodium: 0 mg; Fiber: 5.4 g; Carbs.: 34.2 g; Sugar: 3.2 g; Zinc: 1.3 mg; Calcium: 48.3 mg; Iron: 2.5 mg; Vit. D: 0 mcg; Vit. B_{12}: 0 mcg

Quick and Easy Vegan Biscuits

Use these multipurpose vegan biscuits to mop up your vegetarian gravy, or top with vegan margarine or jam, pour some Earl Grey, and enjoy a British afternoon tea.
Yields 14 biscuits

2 c. flour	½ t. salt
3 t. baking powder	5 T. cold vegan margarine
½ t. onion powder	⅔ c. unsweetened soy milk
½ t. garlic powder	

1. Preheat oven to 425°F.
2. Combine flour, baking powder, onion powder, garlic powder, and salt in a large bowl. Add margarine.
3. Using a fork, mash the margarine with the dry ingredients until crumbly.
4. Add soy milk a few tablespoons at a time and combine just until dough forms. You may need to add a little more or less than ⅔ cup.
5. Knead a few times on a floured surface, then roll out to ¾ inch thick. Cut into 3-inch rounds.
6. Bake for 12–14 minutes, or until done.

It's Great to Be Vegan! Summer is a wonderful time for vegans. Not only is it great for fresh produce, but it's also the season for festivals and fairs! Most major cities have a summer vegetarian festival, which is sure to be packed with lots of great food, speakers, fun, and lots of other vegans. Find out when there's a vegetarian or Earth Day festival near you and add it to your calendar.

Saturday

Glasses of Water Consumed: _____

Thoughts About Today: _____

_____

_____

What I Ate Today

Time	Food Item	Amount	Calories	Fat	Carbs	Fiber	Protein
TOTAL							

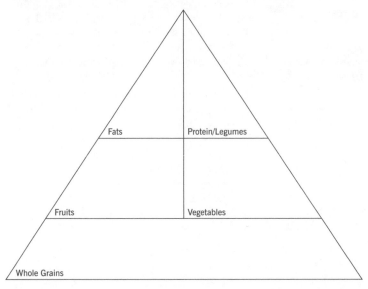

Sunday

Breakfast

2 Morning Cereal Bars

Cal.: 572; Fat: 28 g; Protein: 15.4 g; Sodium: 202 mg; Fiber: 8.6 g; Carbs.: 84 g; Sugar: 48 g; Zinc: 5.2 mg; Calcium: 110 mg; Iron: 8.6 mg; Vit. D: 24 mcg; Vit. B$_{12}$: 1.74 mcg

Lunch

1 Easy Vegan Pizza Bagel (see recipe in Week 1, Wed.), Greek spinach salad with 2 c. fresh spinach, ½ red bell pepper, 2 T. black olives, ¼ c. chopped artichoke hearts, and 2 T. Goddess Dressing (see recipe in Week 1, Mon.)

Cal.: 509; Fat: 17.6 g; Protein: 18.4 g; Sodium: 1173 mg; Fiber: 10.12 g; Carbs.: 78.2 g; Sugar: 7.36 g; Zinc: 1.58 mg; Calcium: 139 mg; Iron: 9.22 mg; Vit. D: 1 mcg; Vit. B$_{12}$: 0 mcg

Snack

2 leftover Quick and Easy Vegan Biscuits (see recipe in Week 8, Sat.), 2 T. sugar-free jam

Cal.: 224; Fat: 8.8 g; Protein: 4.4 g; Sodium: 178 mg; Fiber: 1.12 g; Carbs.: 35 g; Sugar: 0 g; Zinc: 0.44 mg; Calcium: 136 mg; Iron: 2.2 mg; Vit. D: 0 mcg; Vit. B$_{12}$: 0.3 mcg

Dinner

1 c. Chinese Fried Rice with Tofu and Cashews, 1 c. pineapple

Cal.: 387.83; Fat: 18.87 g; Protein: 16.23 g; Sodium: 689.7 mg; Fiber: 4.97 g; Carbs.: 44.27 g; Sugar: 16.607 g; Zinc: 1.73 mg; Calcium: 529.5 mg; Iron: 3.77 mg; Vit. D: 0 mcg; Vit. B$_{12}$: 0 mcg

Morning Cereal Bars

Store-bought breakfast bars are often loaded with artificial sugars, and most homemade recipes require corn syrup. This healthier method makes a sweet and filling snack or breakfast to munch on the run. **Yields 14 bars**

3 c. breakfast cereal, any kind	½ t. vanilla
1 c. peanut butter	2 c. muesli
⅓ c. tahini	½ c. flax meal or wheat germ
1 c. maple syrup	½ c. diced dried fruit or raisins

1. Lightly grease a baking pan or two casserole pans.
2. Place cereal in a sealable bag and crush partially with a rolling pin. If you're using a smaller cereal, you can skip this step. Set aside.
3. Combine peanut butter, tahini, and maple syrup in a large saucepan over low heat, stirring well to combine.
4. Remove from heat and stir in the vanilla, and then the cereal, muesli, flax meal or wheat germ, and dried fruit or raisins.
5. Press firmly into greased baking pan and chill until firm, about 45 minutes, then slice into bars.

Chinese Fried Rice with Tofu and Cashews

On busy weeknights, pick up some plain white rice from a Chinese take-out restaurant and turn it into a home-cooked meal in a jiffy. Garnish with fresh lime wedges and a sprinkle of sea salt and fresh black pepper on top. **Serves 3**

2 cloves garlic, minced	3 T. soy sauce
1 (12-oz.) block silken tofu, mashed with a fork	1 T. sesame oil
3 T. olive oil (divided)	2 T. lime juice
3 c. leftover rice	3 scallions (greens and whites), sliced
½ c. frozen mixed diced veggies	⅓ c. chopped cashews (optional)

1. In a large skillet or wok, sauté the garlic and tofu in 2 tablespoons of olive oil over medium high heat, stirring frequently, until tofu is lightly browned, about 6–8 minutes.
2. Add remaining 1 tablespoon of olive oil, rice, and veggies, stirring well to combine.
3. Add soy sauce and sesame oil and combine well.
4. Allow to cook, stirring constantly, for 3–4 minutes.
5. Remove from heat and stir in remaining ingredients.

Date ____ / ____ / ____

Glasses of Water Consumed: _____

Thoughts About Today: _____

_____

_____

What I Ate Today

Time	Food Item	Amount	Calories	Fat	Carbs	Fiber	Protein
TOTAL							

Fats

Protein/Legumes

Fruits

Vegetables

Whole Grains

Is Your Soy Cheese Vegan?
Many nondairy products do actually contain dairy, even if it says "nondairy" right there on the package! Nondairy creamer and soy cheeses are notorious for this. Look for *casein* or *whey* on the ingredients list, particularly if you suffer from dairy allergies, and, if you're allergic to soy, look for nut- or rice-based vegan cheeses.

WEEK 8 IN REVIEW

I feel: _____
_____
_____
_____

My greatest food discovery this week was: _____
_____
_____
_____

This week's biggest vegan challenge was: _____
_____
_____
_____

New food I'd like to try: _____
_____
_____
_____

When I look back at this week, I most want to remember: ___
_____
_____
_____

Nutrition Totals

	Calories	Fat	Carbs	Fiber	Protein
Goal					
Actual					

WEEK 9

You've come a long way, and you have likely experienced a few ups and downs along the journey. Soon you'll be planning meals on your own, but this week, you've got nothing to worry about at all. Just enjoy the ride, carefree and breezy.

If you have some spare time this week, stop by and browse through a few ethnic restaurants in your neighborhood or near your workplace. Pick up a menu, if you can, and take it home to browse for vegan items. Keep an eye out for Japanese, Thai, Chinese, Mediterranean, and Indian places, or stop by a couple of sandwich shops to see what options they have for vegetarians, minus the cheese and mayonnaise, of course. Make a list of vegan options for when you're ready to start eating out.

Monday

Breakfast

2 Morning Cereal Bars (see recipe in Week 8, Sun.), 1 c. orange juice

Cal.: 396; Fat: 13 g; Protein: 9.7 g; Sodium: 101 mg; Fiber: 4.3 g; Carbs.: 68 g; Sugar: 46 g; Zinc: 2.6 mg; Calcium: 405 mg; Iron: 6.55 mg; Vit. D: 12 mcg; Vit. B_{12}: 1.28 mcg

Lunch

Sandwich with 1 oz. Sun-Dried Tomato Pesto (see recipe in Week 2, Mon.), 1 oz. avocado, ¼ medium tomato, and 1 c. sprouts on 2 slices whole grain bread

Cal.: 427.53; Fat: 14.35 g; Protein: 16.88 g; Sodium: 610.55 mg; Fiber: 9.18 g; Carbs.: 61.2 g; Sugar: 31.4 g; Zinc: 1.05 mg; Calcium: 432.68 mg; Iron: 2.68 mg; Vit. D: 0 mcg; Vit. B_{12}: 0.41 mcg

Snack

Mixed veggies (½ cucumber, 2 oz. baby carrots, ½ c. broccoli) with 2 T. hummus

Cal.: 116.92; Fat: 3.32 g; Protein: 5.38 g; Sodium: 189.5 mg; Fiber: 6.52 g; Carbs.: 19.37 g; Sugar: 6.12 g; Zinc: 1.27 mg; Calcium: 81.63 mg; Iron: 2.18 mg; Vit. D: 0 mcg; Vit. B_{12}: 0 mcg

Dinner

5 oz. Asian Sesame Tahini Noodles (see recipe in Week 1, Sat.)

Cal.: 396; Fat: 12 g; Protein: 15 g; Sodium: 952 mg; Fiber: 2.6 g; Carbs.: 65 g; Sugar: 0.26 g; Zinc: 2.5 mg; Calcium: 118 mg; Iron: 3.3 mg; Vit. D: 0 mcg; Vit. B_{12}: 0 mcg

Don't Get Bored of Bread! Exploring a few quality gourmet ingredients can really perk up your vegan diet if you're in a rut. Use an artisan bread to make sandwiches more satisfying, and leave the regular stuff for morning toast. Try ciabatta rolls, foccaccia, or try something new from your local bakery.

Date ____ / ____ / ____

Glasses of Water Consumed: _____

Thoughts About Today: _____

_____

_____

What I Ate Today

Time	Food Item	Amount	Calories	Fat	Carbs	Fiber	Protein
TOTAL							

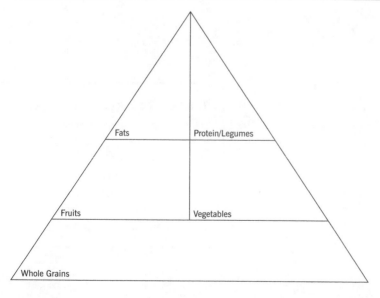

Tuesday

Breakfast

1 c. instant grits with 1 (1-oz.) slice vegan cheese, 1 c. applesauce

Cal.: 285; Fat: 2.7 g; Protein: 4.8 g; Sodium: 664.9 mg; Fiber: 3.4 g; Carbs.: 63.6 g; Sugar: 23.1 g; Zinc: 0.3 mg; Calcium: 217.1 mg; Iron: 2.1 mg; Vit. D: 0 mcg; Vit. B_{12}: 0 mcg

Lunch

1 baked potato with ½ c. black beans, salsa, vegan cheese, side green salad with 2 c. romaine lettuce, 1 tomato, and 1 diced cucumber, 2 T. Goddess Dressing (see recipe in Week 1, Mon.)

Cal.: 434.6; Fat: 13.2 g; Protein: 14 g; Sodium: 591.2 mg; Fiber: 10.12 g; Carbs.: 102.5 g; Sugar: 44.36 g; Zinc: 2.18 mg; Calcium: 652.6 mg; Iron: 15.62 mg; Vit. D: 0 mcg; Vit. B_{12}: 0.41 mcg

Snack

2 Morning Cereal Bars (see recipe in Week 8, Sun.), 1 c. strawberries

Cal.: 620.6; Fat: 26.5 g; Protein: 16.4 g; Sodium: 203.5 mg; Fiber: 11.6 g; Carbs.: 95.7 g; Sugar: 55.4 g; Zinc: 5.4 mg; Calcium: 134.3 mg; Iron: 9.2 mg; Vit. D: 24 mcg; Vit. B_{12}: 1.74 mcg

Dinner

4 oz. Lazy and Hungry Garlic Pasta with 1 tomato, diced

Cal.: 474.1; Fat: 15.2 g; Protein: 17.1 g; Sodium: 642.2 mg; Fiber: 5.1 g; Carbs.: 70.8 g; Sugar: 4.7 g; Zinc: 0.58 mg; Calcium: 33.3 mg; Iron: 4.2 mg; Vit. D: 0 mcg; Vit. B_{12}: 0.18 mcg

Lazy and Hungry Garlic Pasta

Serves 6

2 cloves garlic, minced

2 tablespoons olive oil

3 cups pasta, cooked

2 tablespoons nutritional yeast

½ teaspoon parsley

Dash red pepper flakes (optional)

Salt and pepper to taste

1. Heat the garlic in olive oil for just a minute or two until almost browned.
2. Toss garlic and olive oil with remaining ingredients. Adjust seasonings to taste.

The Perfect Vegan Flavor Mix?

Garlic powder, nutritional yeast, and salt is a delicious seasoning combination, and will give you a bit of a B_{12} perk-up. Perfect for vegans. Use it over toast, veggies, popcorn, bagels, baked potatoes, and, of course, cooked pasta, if you're feeling, well, lazy and hungry!

Glasses of Water Consumed: _____

Thoughts About Today: _____

_____

_____

What I Ate Today

Time	Food Item	Amount	Calories	Fat	Carbs	Fiber	Protein
TOTAL							

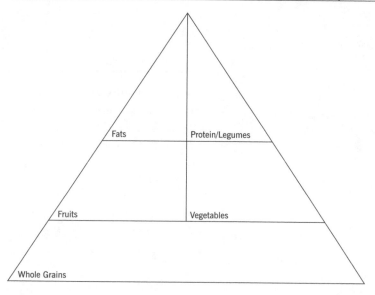

Fats   Protein/Legumes

Fruits   Vegetables

Whole Grains

Wednesday

Breakfast

1 c. whole grain cereal with ½ c. soy milk

Cal.: 178.33; Fat: 2.92 g; Protein: 6.17 g; Sodium: 267.83 mg; Fiber: 4.6 g; Carbs.: 33.43 g; Sugar: 7.17 g; Zinc: 20 mg; Calcium: 1373.33 mg; Iron: 247.7 mg; Vit. D: 54.7 mcg; Vit. B$_{12}$: 8.18 mcg

Lunch

1 vegan grilled cheese sandwich with 2 (1-oz.) slices vegan cheese on 2 slices whole grain bread, tomato soup (about 150 calories), 1 small apple

Record nutritional values for your choice of tomato soup in today's journal. The nutritional values below are for vegan grilled cheese sandwich and apple.

Cal.: 295; Fat: 6.5 g; Protein: 9.4 g; Sodium: 461.5 mg; Fiber: 7.4 g; Carbs.: 53.2 g; Sugar: 18.9 g; Zinc: 0.9 mg; Calcium: 462.1 mg; Iron: 1.6 mg; Vit. D: 0 mcg; Vit. B$_{12}$: 0 mcg

Snack

1 rice cake with 1 T. almond butter

Cal.: 211; Fat: 10.7 g; Protein: 4.4 g; Sodium: 21.7 mg; Fiber: 1.8 g; Carbs.: 26.1 g; Sugar: 0.2 g; Zinc: 1.3 mg; Calcium: 46.3 mg; Iron: 1 mg; Vit. D: 0 mcg; Vit. B$_{12}$: 0 mcg

Dinner

5 oz. Basic Baked Tempeh Patties, 1 c. steamed cauliflower, 1 medium baked sweet potato

Cal.: 360; Fat: 17.2 g; Protein: 28.2 g; Sodium: 1207 mg; Fiber: 4.85 g; Carbs.: 30.7 g; Sugar: 6.88 g; Zinc: 1.7 mg; Calcium: 183.8 mg; Iron: 4.8 mg; Vit. D: 0 mcg; Vit. B$_{12}$: 0 mcg

Basic Baked Tempeh Patties

Baked tempeh is a simple entrée, or use as a patty to make veggie burgers or sandwiches. Slice your tempeh into cubes to add to fried rice, noodles, or stir-fries.
Serves 2

1 (8-oz.) package tempeh
1 c. + 2 T. water or vegetable broth
3 T. soy sauce
2 T. apple cider vinegar
3 cloves garlic, minced
2 t. sesame oil

1. If your tempeh is thicker than ¾ inch, slice in half through the center to make two thinner pieces, then cut into desired shapes.
2. Simmer tempeh in 1 cup water or vegetable broth for 10 minutes; drain well.
3. Whisk together remaining ingredients, including 2 tablespoons of water or vegetable broth, and marinate tempeh for at least 1 hour or overnight.
4. Preheat oven to 375°F and transfer tempeh to a lightly greased baking sheet.
5. Bake for 10–12 minutes on each side.

Using "Planned-Overs" Cooked whole grains can stretch out just about any meal to add some healthy fiber and a touch of homemade goodness to canned chili and soup, baked beans, even green salads or bean salads. Whenever you cook grains, cook a cup or so extra and store them in a tightly sealed container in the refrigerator.

Glasses of Water Consumed: _____

Thoughts About Today: _____

_____

_____

What I Ate Today

Time	Food Item	Amount	Calories	Fat	Carbs	Fiber	Protein
TOTAL							

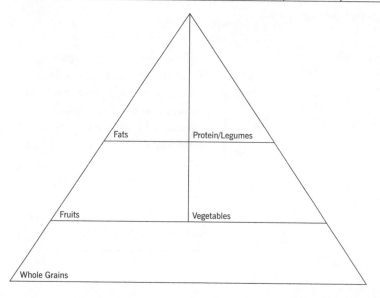

Fats   Protein/Legumes

Fruits   Vegetables

Whole Grains

Thursday

Breakfast

1 bagel with 2 T. hummus, 1 c. soy milk

Cal.: 286; Fat: 8.2 g; Protein: 15.1 g; Sodium: 397.6 mg; Fiber: 5.1 g; Carbs.: 38.2 g; Sugar: 3.9 g; Zinc: 1.7 mg; Calcium: 142.1 mg; Iron: 5.6 mg; Vit. D: 3 mcg; Vit. B_{12}: 0.36 mcg

Lunch

Eggless Egg Salad (see recipe in Week 4, Mon.) sandwich with ¼ tomato, sliced, and ¼ c. romaine lettuce on 2 slices whole grain bread

Cal.: 318.73; Fat: 14.25 g; Protein: 18.28 g; Sodium: 502.55 mg; Fiber: 5.88 g; Carbs.: 32.5 g; Sugar: 7.2 g; Zinc: 2.05 mg; Calcium: 444.28 mg; Iron: 3.48 mg; Vit. D: 0 mcg; Vit. B_{12}: 0 mcg

Snack

Mixed fruit salad with ½ apple, ½ banana, ½ c. strawberries, and ½ c. pineapple, 1 oz. raisins

Cal.: 233.75; Fat: 0.75 g; Protein: 2.6 g; Sodium: 5.95 mg; Fiber: 6.75 g; Carbs.: 60.9 g; Sugar: 42.5 g; Zinc: 0.45 mg; Calcium: 44 mg; Iron: 1.3 mg; Vit. D: 0 mcg; Vit. B_{12}: 0 mcg

Dinner

9¼ oz. Eggplant Baba Ganoush, 1 pita, and Greek spinach salad (2 c. fresh spinach, ½ red bell pepper, 2 T. black olives, ¼ c. chopped artichoke hearts) with 2 T. Goddess Dressing (see recipe in Week 1, Mon.)

Cal.: 437; Fat: 32.6 g; Protein: 10.5 g; Sodium: 557 mg; Fiber: 13.32 g; Carbs.: 36.2 g; Sugar: 9.06 g; Zinc: 1.35 mg; Calcium: 211 mg; Iron: 5.81 mg; Vit. D: 0 mcg; Vit. B_{12}: 0 mcg

Eggplant Baba Ganoush

Serves 4

2 medium eggplants
3 T. olive oil, divided
2 T. lemon juice
¼ c. tahini
3 cloves garlic

½ t. cumin
½ t. chili powder (optional)
¼ t. salt
1 T. chopped fresh parsley

1. Preheat oven to 400°F. Slice eggplants in half and prick several times with a fork.
2. Place on a baking sheet and drizzle with 1 T. olive oil. Bake for 30 minutes, or until soft. Allow to cool slightly.
3. Remove inner flesh and place in a bowl.
4. Using a large fork or potato masher, mash eggplant together with remaining ingredients until almost smooth.
5. Adjust seasonings to taste.

Halfway Homemade Vegan Meals Shop the ethnic food aisle or bulk section for lots of mixes that can be prepared at home in an instant. Tabouli, hummus, and falafel mixes and even veggie burger mixes are a great thing to keep on hand. Just add water or olive oil, and they're ready to go. To freshen them up a bit, mix a few fresh tomatoes into a tabouli mix, or add in some sliced olives or cumin to a hummus mix.

Thursday

Glasses of Water Consumed: _____

Thoughts About Today: _____

_____

_____

What I Ate Today

Time	Food Item	Amount	Calories	Fat	Carbs	Fiber	Protein
TOTAL							

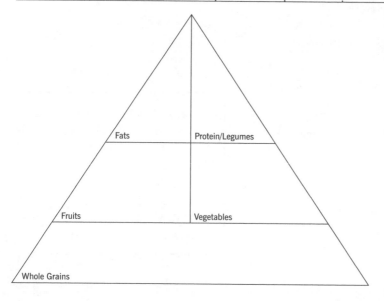

Friday

Breakfast

1 c. baked beans, 2 slices whole grain toast, 1 small banana, 1 c. chocolate soy milk

Cal.: 386.6; Fat: 4.4 g; Protein: 14.9 g; Sodium: 731.5 mg; Fiber: 14.5 g; Carbs.: 74.9 g; Sugar: 42.2 g; Zinc: 3.2 mg; Calcium: 375.5 mg; Iron: 4.68 mg; Vit. D: 0 mcg; Vit. B$_{12}$: 0 mcg

Lunch

9¼ oz. leftover Eggplant Baba Ganoush (see recipe in Week 9, Thurs.), 1 pita, side green salad with 2 c. romaine lettuce, 1 tomato, and 1 diced cucumber, 2 T. Goddess Dressing (see recipe in Week 1, Mon.), 1 c. tomato juice

Cal.: 643; Fat: 31.1 g; Protein: 18.9 g; Sodium: 734.5 mg; Fiber: 16.62 g; Carbs.: 84.6 g; Sugar: 23.86 g; Zinc: 3.25 mg; Calcium: 307.4 mg; Iron: 6.51 mg; Vit. D: 0 mcg; Vit. B$_{12}$: 0 mcg

Snack

1 small apple, 1 T. peanut butter, 1 oz. raisins

Cal.: 169.35; Fat: 4.35 g; Protein: 3.35 g; Sodium: 4.55 mg; Fiber: 4.6 g; Carbs.: 33.2 g; Sugar: 24.3 g; Zinc: 0.15 mg; Calcium: 15.9 mg; Iron: 0.45 mg; Vit. D: 0 mcg; Vit. B$_{12}$: 0 mcg

Dinner

Veggie chicken burger with 1 vegan chicken patty, ¼ tomato, sliced, and 12.5 oz. Sesame and Soy Cole Slaw Salad

Cal.: 391; Fat: 20 g; Protein: 11.7 g; Sodium: 401 mg; Fiber: 5 g; Carbs.: 44 g; Sugar: 16 g; Zinc: 8.4 mg; Calcium: 97 mg; Iron: 2.9 mg; Vit. D: 0 mcg; Vit. B$_{12}$: 0 mcg

Sesame and Soy Cole Slaw Salad

Serves 2

1 head Napa cabbage, shredded

1 carrot, grated

2 green onions, chopped

1 red bell pepper, sliced thin

2 T. olive oil

2 T. apple cider vinegar

2 t. soy sauce

½ t. sesame oil

2 T. maple syrup

2 T. sesame seeds (optional)

1. Toss together cabbage, carrot, green onions, and bell pepper in a large bowl.
2. In a separate small bowl, whisk together the olive oil, vinegar, soy sauce, sesame oil, and maple syrup until well combined.
3. Drizzle dressing over cabbage and veggies, add sesame seeds, and toss well to combine.

Mideast Treats Middle-Eastern restaurants are always a safe bet for vegans eating out. You're pretty much guaranteed to find vegan falafel, hummus, baba ganoush, fattoush, and those absolutely divine stuffed grape leaves. The best part? They're all vegan already! No need to ask a server to hold the cheese.

Glasses of Water Consumed: _____

Thoughts About Today: _____

_____

_____

What I Ate Today

Time	Food Item	Amount	Calories	Fat	Carbs	Fiber	Protein
TOTAL							

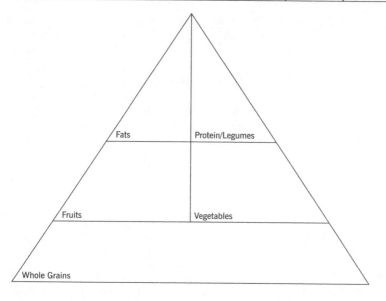

Saturday

Breakfast

3 slices Easy Vegan French Toast (see recipe in Week 1, Sun.), 1 c. fresh strawberries, 1 c. orange juice

Cal.: 473.6; Fat: 4.1 g; Protein: 13 g; Sodium: 429.5 mg; Fiber: 11 g; Carbs.: 100.7 g; Sugar: 50.4 g; Zinc: 1.6 mg; Calcium: 512.6 mg; Iron: 5.75 mg; Vit. D: 0 mcg; Vit. B$_{12}$: 0.84 mcg

Lunch

3 oz. Lemon Quinoa Veggie Salad

Cal.: 262; Fat: 12 g; Protein: 6.6 g; Sodium: 221 mg; Fiber: 4.1 g; Carbs.: 34 g; Sugar: 0 g; Zinc: 1.3 mg; Calcium: 35 mg; Iron: 4.3 mg; Vit. D: 0 mcg; Vit. B$_{12}$: 0 mcg

Snack

1 c. edamame

Cal.: 189; Fat: 8.1 g; Protein: 16.9 g; Sodium: 9.3 mg; Fiber: 8.1 g; Carbs.: 15.8 g; Sugar: 3.4 g; Zinc: 2.1 mg; Calcium: 97.6 mg; Iron: 3.5 mg; Vit. D: 0 mcg; Vit. B$_{12}$: 0 mcg

Dinner

12 oz. Polenta and Chili Casserole, 1 c. steamed spinach with 16 g nutritional yeast

Cal.: 443.4; Fat: 6.7 g; Protein: 29.3 g; Sodium: 846 mg; Fiber: 22.3 g; Carbs.: 73.7 g; Sugar: 9.3 g; Zinc: 7.1 mg; Calcium: 357 mg; Iron: 10.3 mg; Vit. D: 0 mcg; Vit. B$_{12}$: 7.8 mcg

Lemon Quinoa Veggie Salad

Serves 6

1½ c. quinoa	1 t. garlic powder
4 c. vegetable broth	½ t. sea salt
1 c. frozen mixed veggies, thawed	¼ t. black pepper
¼ c. lemon juice	2 T. chopped fresh cilantro or parsley (optional)
¼ c. olive oil	

1. In a large pot, simmer quinoa in vegetable broth for 15–20 minutes, stirring occasionally, until liquid is absorbed and quinoa is cooked. Add mixed veggies and stir to combine.
2. Remove from heat and combine with remaining ingredients. Serve hot or cold.

Polenta and Chile Casserole

Using canned chili and thawed frozen veggies, you can get this quick one-pot casserole meal in the oven in just about ten minutes. **Serves 6**

3 (14.7 oz.) cans vegetarian chili (or about 6 c. homemade)	1 c. cornmeal
	2½ c. water
2 c. diced veggie mixture, any kind	2 T. vegan margarine
	1 T. chili powder

1. Combine vegetarian chili and vegetables, and spread in the bottom of a lightly greased casserole dish.
2. Preheat oven to 375°F.
3. Over low heat, combine cornmeal and water. Simmer, stirring frequently, for 10 minutes. Stir in vegan margarine.
4. Spread cornmeal mixture over chili and sprinkle the top with chili powder.
5. Bake uncovered for 20–25 minutes.

Glasses of Water Consumed: _____

Thoughts About Today: _____

_____

_____

What I Ate Today

Time	Food Item	Amount	Calories	Fat	Carbs	Fiber	Protein
TOTAL							

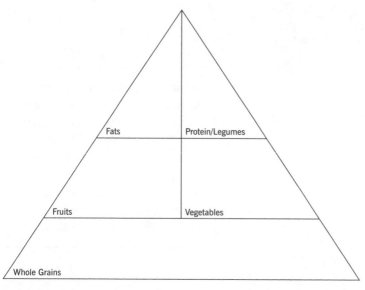

Fats

Protein/Legumes

Fruits

Vegetables

Whole Grains

Sunday

Breakfast

1 c. Pumpkin Protein Smoothie (see recipe in Week 3, Thurs.), 1 banana, 1 oz. cashews

Cal.: 371.9; Fat: 15.4 g; Protein: 11.6 g; Sodium: 67.4 mg; Fiber: 5.5 g; Carbs.: 53.3 g; Sugar: 22.8 g; Zinc: 2.56 mg; Calcium: 260.5 mg; Iron: 4.1 mg; Vit. D: 0 mcg; Vit. B_{12}: 1.5 mcg

Lunch

Bean burrito with ½ c. beef substitute, 1 flour tortilla, ½ tomato, sliced, and ½ c. iceberg lettuce

Cal.: 387.1; Fat: 5.5 g; Protein: 22.85 g; Sodium: 952.7 mg; Fiber: 13 g; Carbs.: 55.5 g; Sugar: 7.3 g; Zinc: 1.85 mg; Calcium: 104.65 mg; Iron: 3.9 mg; Vit. D: 0 mcg; Vit. B_{12}: 0 mcg

Snack

1 Peanut Butter Rice Crispie

Cal.: 427; Fat: 16 g; Protein: 8.1 g; Sodium: 140 mg; Fiber: 1.4 g; Carbs.: 66 g; Sugar: 5.1 g; Zinc: 0.79 mg; Calcium: 30 mg; Iron: 1.5 mg; Vit. D: 0 mcg; Vit. B_{12}: 0.81 mcg

Dinner

¼ block Easy Barbecue Baked Tofu (see recipe in Week 2, Wed.), 1 c. Caramelized Baby Carrots (see recipe in Week 1, Tues.), 1 ear corn on the cob

Cal.: 537; Fat: 18.5 g; Protein: 20.5 g; Sodium: 817 mg; Fiber: 5.6 g; Carbs.: 83.2 g; Sugar: 35.6 g; Zinc: 2.5 mg; Calcium: 628.73 mg; Iron: 5.43 mg; Vit. D: 0 mcg; Vit. B_{12}: .01 mcg

Peanut Butter Rice Crispies

Serves 9

¾ c. sugar
¾ c. golden syrup
¾ c. peanut butter
4½ c. rice crispie cereal
⅔ c. chocolate chips

1. Lightly grease a 9" × 9" baking dish.
2. Heat the sugar and golden syrup on the stove top just until simmering. Remove from heat and stir in peanut butter until well combined, then gently stir in cereal and chocolate chips.
3. Spread mixture evenly into baking pan, using a large spoon or spatula to flatten. Chill in the refrigerator until firm, then slice into squares.

Honey: To Bee or Not to Bee?

Many vegans assume honey is cruelty-free and gently collected from bees that are producing it naturally. This is simply not true. Though the subject is often debated among vegans, according to the manifesto set forth by the British Vegan Society in 1944, honey is an animal by-product and therefore not vegan.

Glasses of Water Consumed: _____

Thoughts About Today: _____

_____

_____

What I Ate Today

Time	Food Item	Amount	Calories	Fat	Carbs	Fiber	Protein
TOTAL							

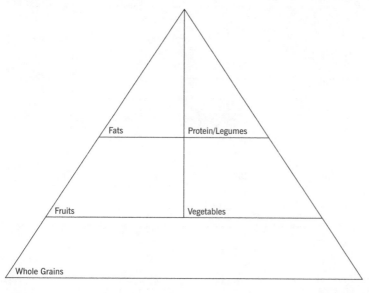

WEEK 9 IN REVIEW

I feel: _____
_____
_____
_____

My greatest food discovery this week was: _____
_____
_____
_____

This week's biggest vegan challenge was: _____
_____
_____
_____

New food I'd like to try: _____
_____
_____
_____

When I look back at this week, I most want to remember: _____
_____
_____
_____

Nutrition Totals

	Calories	Fat	Carbs	Fiber	Protein
Goal					
Actual					

WEEK 10

Start planning how you'll be eating after these twelve weeks are up. Are there some meals that you loved and will continue eating every week? Or perhaps you never want to touch tempeh ever again! Identify a few convenience foods that will keep you well stocked and well fed under any circumstances. Start collecting a few recipes that you'd like to try once you're on your own, and maybe even plan a few complete meals to have on deck ready to go for week thirteen. Meals don't have to be complex to be nutritious. Think of a few things you can make easily, without a recipe. Chickpeas with a few tomatoes and Indian spices paired with quinoa can be on your plate in minutes. Beans can be simmered with chili powder and paired with rice and veggies. A huge vegetable salad is always delicious and easy to make. Think you can whip up some vegan burritos, tacos, soups, and tofu dishes without a recipe?

Review your notes from the past weeks, and think about some of the meals that you enjoyed and were easy enough to prepare on busy weeknights. You'll need them soon, when you're on your own!

Of course, if you really don't want to think about things, you could always start this meal plan all over at the beginning!

Monday

Breakfast

12 oz. Chocolate Peanut Butter Banana Smoothie (see recipe in Week 1, Thurs.)

Cal.: 288; Fat: 11 g; Protein: 10 g; Sodium: 124 mg; Fiber: 7 g; Carbs.: 45 g; Sugar: 20 g; Zinc: 1.1 mg; Calcium: 205 mg; Iron: 1.8 mg; Vit. D: 0 mcg; Vit. B$_{12}$: 1.5 mcg

Snack

1 Peanut Butter Rice Crispie (see recipe in Week 9, Sun.)

Cal.: 427; Fat: 16 g; Protein: 8.1 g; Sodium: 140 mg; Fiber: 1.4 g; Carbs.: 66 g; Sugar: 5.1 g; Zinc: 0.79 mg; Calcium: 30 mg; Iron: 1.5 mg; Vit. D: 0 mcg; Vit. B$_{12}$: 0.81 mcg

Lunch

Barbecue tofu sandwiches with ¼ block leftover Easy Barbecue Baked Tofu (see recipe in Week 2, Wed.), ¼ tomato, ¼ c. iceberg lettuce, and 1 T. vegan mayonnaise on 2 slices whole wheat bread, 1 small apple

Cal.: 400.65; Fat: 12.38 g; Protein: 18.33 g; Sodium: 643.85 mg; Fiber: 7.7 g; Carbs.: 59.68 g; Sugar: 35.35 g; Zinc: 2.18 mg; Calcium: 592.83 mg; Iron: 3.45 mg; Vit. D: 0 mcg; Vit. B$_{12}$: 0 mcg

Dinner

10½ oz. Winter Seitan Stew, 1 c. steamed cauliflower with 16 g nutritional yeast, side green salad with 2 c. romaine lettuce, 1 tomato, and 1 diced cucumber, 2 T. Goddess Dressing (see recipe in Week 1, Mon.)

Cal.: 658.7; Fat: 29.4 g; Protein: 36 g; Sodium: 312.2 mg; Fiber: 17.5 g; Carbs.: 75.7 g; Sugar: 16.91 g; Zinc: 5.72 mg; Calcium: 300.5 mg; Iron: 8.47 mg; Vit. D: 0 mcg; Vit. B$_{12}$: 7.8 mcg

Winter Seitan Stew

If you're used to a "meat and potatoes" kind of diet, this hearty seitan and potato stew ought to become a favorite. **Serves 6**

2 c. chopped seitan	½ t. sage
1 onion, chopped	½ t. rosemary
2 carrots, chopped	½ t. thyme
2 ribs celery, chopped	2 T. cornstarch
2 T. olive oil	⅓ c. water
4 c. vegetable broth	Salt and pepper to taste
2 potatoes, chopped	

1. In a large soup pot, heat seitan, onion, carrots, and celery in olive oil, for 4–5 minutes, stirring frequently, until seitan is lightly browned.
2. Add vegetable broth and potatoes and bring to a boil. Reduce to a simmer, add spices and cover. Allow to cook for 25–30 minutes, until potatoes are soft.
3. In a small bowl, whisk together cornstarch and water. Add to soup, stirring to combine.
4. Cook, uncovered, for another 5–7 minutes, until stew has thickened.
5. Season generously with salt and pepper to taste.

What Are Animal Rights? Philosophers Jeremy Bentham and Peter Singer have both written about dominance, use, and exploitation of one being (animals) by another (humans) as a reason to reject animal foods. Agree or disagree, the words of novelist, feminist, and vegan Alice Walker summarize this sentiment: "The animals of the world exist for their own reasons. They were not made for humans any more than black people were made for white, or women created for men." This is the idea of animal rights, that animals may lead their own lives, completely unencumbered by humans.

Glasses of Water Consumed: _____

Thoughts About Today: _____

_____

_____

What I Ate Today

Time	Food Item	Amount	Calories	Fat	Carbs	Fiber	Protein
TOTAL							

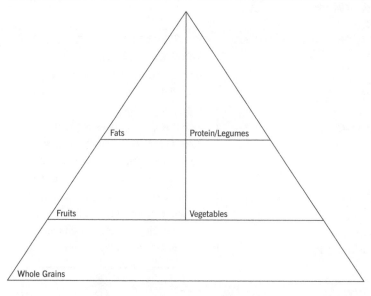

Fats

Protein/Legumes

Fruits

Vegetables

Whole Grains

Breakfast

1 c. oatmeal with 2 t. maple syrup, 1 oz. pecans, 1 c. blueberries

Cal.: 462.33; **Fat**: 24 g; **Protein**: 8.7 g; **Sodium**: 2.7 mg; **Fiber**: 10.3 g; **Carbs.**: 61.26 g; **Sugar**: 25.29 g; **Zinc**: 2.05 mg; **Calcium**: 37.43 mg; **Iron**: 2.06 mg; **Vit. D**: 0 mcg; **Vit. B**$_{12}$: 0 mcg

Lunch

7 oz. leftover Winter Seitan Stew (see recipe in Week 10, Mon.), 1 slice whole grain toast, 1 c. orange juice

Cal.: 564.6; **Fat**: 17.6 g; **Protein**: 25 g; **Sodium**: 191 mg; **Fiber**: 6.85 g; **Carbs.**: 80.8 g; **Sugar**: 27.45 g; **Zinc**: 1.24 mg; **Calcium**: 511.6 mg; **Iron**: 7 mg; **Vit. D**: 0 mcg; **Vit. B**$_{12}$: 0.41 mcg

Snack

Mixed veggies (½ cucumber, 2 oz. baby carrots, ½ c. broccoli) in 2 T. hummus

Cal.: 116.92; **Fat**: 3.32 g; **Protein**: 5.38 g; **Sodium**: 189.5 mg; **Fiber**: 6.52 g; **Carbs.**: 19.37 g; **Sugar**: 6.12 g; **Zinc**: 1.27 mg; **Calcium**: 81.63 mg; **Iron**: 2.18 mg; **Vit. D**: 0 mcg; **Vit. B**$_{12}$: 0 mcg

Dinner

5 oz. Sloppy "Jolindas" with TVP, baked sweet potato, and 16 g nutritional yeast, side green salad with 2 c. romaine lettuce, 1 tomato, and 1 diced cucumber, 2 T. Goddess Dressing (see recipe in Week 1, Mon.)

Cal.: 453.2; **Fat**: 19 g; **Protein**: 25.7 g; **Sodium**: 781.2 mg; **Fiber**: 16.12 g; **Carbs.**: 52.3 g; **Sugar**: 20.36 g; **Zinc**: 8.88 mg; **Calcium**: 239.3 mg; **Iron**: 7.22 mg; **Vit. D**: 2 mcg; **Vit. B**$_{12}$: 7.8 mcg

Sloppy "Jolindas" with TVP

TVP "Sloppy Jolindas" are reminiscent of those goopy sloppy joes served up in primary school cafeterias, with all of the nostalgic comfort and none of the gristle or mystery meat. The TVP is only partially rehydrated, the better to absorb all the flavors. **Serves 8**

1¾ c. TVP	2 T. chili powder
1 c. hot water or vegetable broth	1 T. mustard powder
	1 T. soy sauce
1 onion, chopped	2 T. molasses
1 green bell pepper, chopped small	2 T. apple cider vinegar
2 T. oil	1 t. hot sauce, or to taste
1 (16-oz.) can tomato sauce	1 t. garlic powder
¼ c. barbecue sauce	½ t. salt

1. Combine the TVP and water or vegetable broth and allow to sit at least 5 minutes.

1. In a large soup or stockpot, sauté onion and bell pepper in oil until soft.

2. Reduce heat to medium low and add TVP and remaining ingredients. Simmer, covered, for at least 15 minutes, stirring occasionally.

3. For thicker and less sloppy Sloppy "Jolindas," simmer a bit longer, uncovered, to reduce the liquid.

Yeast Extracts Yeast extracts such as Marmite and Vegemite are more popular abroad than in the United States, and most people tend to either love them or hate them. If you've never tried them, there's only one way to find out how *you* feel! Both are a great source of B vitamins for vegans. Try spreading a bit of yeast extract on your toast, or have a peanut butter and Marmite sandwich! Most people are pretty loyal to one brand or the other, so try them both.

Glasses of Water Consumed: _____

Thoughts About Today: _____

_____

_____

What I Ate Today

Time	Food Item	Amount	Calories	Fat	Carbs	Fiber	Protein
TOTAL							

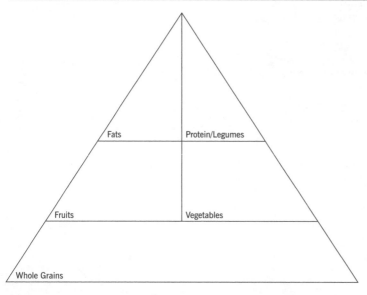

Wednesday

Breakfast

1 pan-fried polenta with ½ c. black beans and 1 (1-oz.) slice vegan cheese, 1 c. soy milk

Cal.: 445.5; Fat: 8.95 g; Protein: 20.2 g; Sodium: 169.45 mg; Fiber: 13.5 g; Carbs.: 73.4 g; Sugar: 1.4 g; Zinc: 1.95 mg; Calcium: 306.6 mg; Iron: 5.2 mg; Vit. D: 3 mcg; Vit. B_{12}: 0.36 mcg

Lunch

Leftover Sloppy "Jolindas" with TVP (see recipe in Week 10, Tues.), side green salad with 2 c. romaine lettuce, 1 tomato, and 1 diced cucumber, 2 T. Goddess Dressing (see recipe in Week 1, Mon.)

Cal.: 354.2; Fat: 18.4 g; Protein: 16.5 g; Sodium: 776.2 mg; Fiber: 10.12 g; Carbs.: 34.9 g; Sugar: 15.46 g; Zinc: 5.68 mg; Calcium: 216.5 mg; Iron: 6.12 mg; Vit. D: 2 mcg; Vit. B_{12}: 0 mcg

Snack

1 c. edamame, 1 c. strawberries

Cal.: 237.6; Fat: 8.6 g; Protein: 17.9 g; Sodium: 10.8 mg; Fiber: 11.1 g; Carbs.: 27.5 g; Sugar: 10.8 g; Zinc: 2.3 mg; Calcium: 121.9 mg; Iron: 4.1 mg; Vit. D: 0 mcg; Vit. B_{12}: 0 mcg

Dinner

6 oz. Spicy Southern Jambalaya, 1 vegan sausage patty, 1 c. steamed spinach

Cal.: 331.4; Fat: 9.7 g; Protein: 20.3 g; Sodium: 105 mg; Fiber: 9.1 g; Carbs.: 43.7 g; Sugar: 2.25 g; Zinc: 1.96 mg; Calcium: 281 mg; Iron: 9.84 mg; Vit. D: 0 mcg; Vit. B_{12}: 2.1 mcg

Spicy Southern Jambalaya

Make this spicy and smoky Southern rice dish a main meal by adding in some browned mock sausage or sautéed tofu. **Serves 6**

1 onion, chopped	1 bay leaf
1 bell pepper, any color, chopped	1 t. paprika
	½ t. thyme
1 rib celery, diced	½ t. oregano
2 T. olive oil	½ t. garlic powder
1 (14-oz.) can diced tomatoes (do not drain)	1 c. corn or frozen mixed diced veggies (optional)
3 c. water or vegetable broth	½ t. cayenne pepper or hot Tabasco sauce to taste
2 c. rice	

1. In a large skillet or stockpot, heat onion, bell pepper, and celery in olive oil until almost soft, about 3 minutes.
2. Reduce heat and add remaining ingredients, except veggies and hot sauce. Cover, bring to a low simmer, and cook for 20 minutes, until rice is done, stirring occasionally.
3. Add veggies and cayenne pepper or hot sauce, and cook just until heated through, about 3 minutes. Adjust seasonings to taste.

Wednesday

Glasses of Water Consumed: _____

Thoughts About Today: _____

_____

_____

What I Ate Today

Time	Food Item	Amount	Calories	Fat	Carbs	Fiber	Protein
TOTAL							

Fats

Protein/Legumes

Fruits

Vegetables

Whole Grains

Leftover Rice Don't let it go to waste! Use leftover rice to make rice and bean burritos, rice salads, or Asian-style fried rice. Add it to soups or pair it with a stir-fry. Leftover plain white rice makes for an excellent rice pudding.

Thursday

Breakfast

1 c. whole grain cereal with ½ c. soy milk, 1 small banana

Cal.: 268.33; Fat: 3.22 g; Protein: 7.27 g; Sodium: 268.83 mg; Fiber: 7.2 g; Carbs.: 56.53 g; Sugar: 19.57 g; Zinc: 20.2 mg; Calcium: 1378.43 mg; Iron: 25 mg; Vit. D: 54.7 mcg; Vit. B$_{12}$: 8.18 mcg

Lunch

6 oz. leftover Spicy Southern Jambalaya (see recipe in Week 10, Wed.) with 1 vegan sausage patty

Cal.: 290; Fat: 9.2 g; Protein: 15 g; Sodium: 105 mg; Fiber: 4.8 g; Carbs.: 37 g; Sugar: 1.45 g; Zinc: 0.56 mg; Calcium: 36 mg; Iron: 3.44 mg; Vit. D: 0 mcg; Vit. B$_{12}$: 2.1 mcg

Snack

200 calories of whole grain crackers with 3 T. olive tapenade

Record nutritional values for your choice of whole grain crackers in today's journal. The nutritional values below are for olive tapenade only.

Cal.: 90; Fat: 6 g; Protein: 0 g; Sodium: 480 mg; Fiber: 0 g; Carbs.: 3 g; Sugar: 0 g; Zinc: 0 mg; Calcium: 69 mg; Iron: 2.1 mg; Vit. D: 0 mcg; Vit. B$_{12}$: 0 mcg

Dinner

6 oz. Tofu BBQ Sauce "Steaks," 4 oz. Baked Sweet Potato Fries (see recipe in Week 4, Thurs.), 1 c. oven-roasted butternut squash

Cal.: 507; Fat: 26.2 g; Protein: 25.8 g; Sodium: 796 mg; Fiber: 5.8 g; Carbs.: 5.1 g; Sugar: 11.5 g; Zinc: 2.9 mg; Calcium: 996 mg; Iron: 6.4 mg; Vit. D: 0 mcg; Vit. B$_{12}$: 0 mcg

Tofu BBQ Sauce "Steaks"

These chewy tofu "steaks" have a hearty texture and a meaty flavor. Delicious as is, or add it to a sandwich. If you've never cooked tofu before, this is a super-easy foolproof recipe to start with. **Serves 5**

⅓ c. barbecue sauce

¼ c. water

2 t. balsamic vinegar

2 T. soy sauce

1–2 T. hot sauce (or to taste)

2 t. sugar

2 blocks firm or extra-firm tofu, well pressed

½ onion, chopped

2 T. olive oil

1. In a small bowl, whisk together the barbecue sauce, water, vinegar, soy sauce, hot sauce, and sugar until well combined. Set aside.
2. Slice pressed tofu into ¼-inch-thick strips.
3. Sauté onions in oil, and carefully add tofu. Fry tofu on both sides until lightly golden brown, about 2 minutes on each side.
4. Reduce heat and add barbecue sauce mixture, stirring to coat tofu well. Cook over medium-low heat until sauce absorbs and thickens, about 5–6 minutes.

Date ____ / ____ / ____

Glasses of Water Consumed: _____

Thoughts About Today: _____

_____

_____

What I Ate Today

Time	Food Item	Amount	Calories	Fat	Carbs	Fiber	Protein
TOTAL							

Tofu, Tempeh, and Seitan This recipe, like many pan-fried or stir-fried tofu recipes, will also work well with seitan or tempeh, though seitan needs a bit longer to cook all the way through; otherwise it ends up tough and chewy.

Fats

Protein/Legumes

Fruits

Vegetables

Whole Grains

Friday

Breakfast

¾ c. Maple Cinnamon Breakfast Quinoa (see recipe in Week 4, Fri.)

Cal.: 421; Fat: 8.4 g; Protein: 14 g; Sodium: 52 mg; Fiber: 5.4 g; Carbs.: 75 g; Sugar: 12 g; Zinc: 3.5 mg; Calcium: 195 mg; Iron: 8.6 mg; Vit. D: 0 mcg; Vit. B$_{12}$: 1 mcg

Lunch

275 calories store-bought vegetarian chili, mixed fruit salad with ½ apple, ½ banana, ½ c. strawberries, and ½ c. pineapple, 1 c. orange juice

Record nutritional values for your choice of vegetarian chili in today's journal. The nutritional values below are for mixed fruit salad and orange juice only.

Cal.: 259.25; Fat: 0.65 g; Protein: 3.7 g; Sodium: 2.85 mg; Fiber: 5.75 g; Carbs.: 64.5 g; Sugar: 47.8 g; Zinc: 0.35 mg; Calcium: 379.9 mg; Iron: 3.05 mg; Vit. D: 0 mcg; Vit. B$_{12}$: 0.41 mcg

Snack

4 oz. leftover Baked Sweet Potato Fries (see recipe in Week 4, Thurs.), 1 oz. peanuts

Cal.: 332; Fat: 23.7 g; Protein: 9.8 g; Sodium: 335.6 mg; Fiber: 5.6 g; Carbs.: 24.3 g; Sugar: 6.2 g; Zinc: 0.9 mg; Calcium: 46.1 mg; Iron: 1.4 mg; Vit. D: 0 mcg; Vit. B$_{12}$: 0 mcg

Dinner

8 oz. Italian Veggie and Pasta Casserole, 1 c. steamed broccoli with 16 g nutritional yeast

Cal.: 506; Fat: 9.7 g; Protein: 25.3 g; Sodium: 288 mg; Fiber: 13.6 g; Carbs.: 87.1 g; Sugar: 4.8 g; Zinc: 4.33 mg; Calcium: 171 mg; Iron: 6 mg; Vit. D: 0 mcg; Vit. B$_{12}$: 7.86 mcg

Italian Veggie and Pasta Casserole

Veggies and pasta are baked into an Italian-spiced casserole with a crumbly topping. Add in a handful of TVP crumbles or some kidney beans if you want a protein boost. **Serves 8**

1 (16-oz.) package pasta (use a medium pasta like bowties, corkscrews, or small shells)	¾ c. corn kernels
	1 t. parsley
	1 t. basil
1 onion, chopped	½ t. oregano
3 zucchinis, sliced	½ t. crushed red pepper flakes
1 red bell pepper, chopped	
4 cloves garlic, minced	¼ t. pepper
2 T. olive oil	1 c. bread crumbs
1 (28-oz.) can diced tomatoes	½ c. grated vegan cheese

1. Cook pasta according to package instructions, drain well, and layer in a baking dish.
2. Preheat oven to 425°F.
3. Sauté onion, zucchini, bell pepper, and garlic in olive oil just until soft, about 3–4 minutes. Add tomatoes, corn, parsley, basil, oregano, and crushed red pepper. Simmer for 8–10 minutes and season with black pepper.
4. Cover pasta with zucchini and tomato mixture. Sprinkle with bread crumbs and vegan cheese.
5. Bake for 10–12 minutes.

Date ____ / ____ / ____

Glasses of Water Consumed: _____

Thoughts About Today: _____

_____

_____

What I Ate Today

Time	Food Item	Amount	Calories	Fat	Carbs	Fiber	Protein
TOTAL							

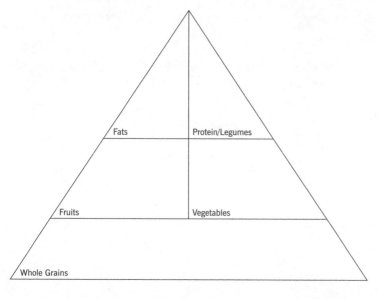

Fats

Protein/Legumes

Fruits

Vegetables

Whole Grains

Saturday

Breakfast

3 Vegan Pancakes (see recipe in Week 3, Sun.),
1 c. fresh strawberries, 1 c. orange juice

Cal.: 410.6; Fat: 2.5 g; Protein: 9 g; Sodium: 231.5 mg;
Fiber: 6 g; Carbs.: 89.7 g; Sugar: 40.4 g; Zinc: 0.62 mg;
Calcium: 632.6 mg; Iron: 5.65 mg; Vit. D: 0 mcg; Vit.
B$_{12}$: 1.41 mcg

Lunch

6 oz. Mexico City Protein Bowl

Cal.: 465; Fat: 9.7 g; Protein: 27 g; Sodium: 113 mg;
Fiber: 15 g; Carbs.: 71 g; Sugar: 2.8 g; Zinc: 4.3 mg;
Calcium: 372 mg; Iron: 5.7 mg; Vit. D: 0 mcg; Vit. B$_{12}$:
0 mcg

Snack

1 c. soy yogurt with ⅓ c. granola

Cal.: 334; Fat: 12.5 g; Protein: 10.2 g; Sodium: 91.1
mg; Fiber: 4.2 g; Carbs.: 51.2 g; Sugar: 26.7 g; Zinc:
1.2 mg; Calcium: 44.7 mg; Iron: 1.4 mg; Vit. D: 0 mcg;
Vit. B$_{12}$: 0 mcg

Dinner

1½ c. Barley Vegetable Soup, side green salad
with 2 c. romaine lettuce, 1 tomato, and 1 diced
cucumber, 2 T. Goddess Dressing (see recipe in
Week 1, Mon.)

Cal.: 512.2; Fat: 21.15 g; Protein: 16.25 g; Sodium:
430.2 mg; Fiber: 19.32 g; Carbs.: 71.4 g; Sugar: 11.23
g; Zinc: 29.75 mg; Calcium: 227.5 mg; Iron: 6.77 mg;
Vit. D: 0 mcg; Vit. B$_{12}$: 0 mcg

Mexico City Protein Bowl

Serves 4

½ block firm tofu, diced small	½ c. corn kernels
1 scallion, chopped	½ t. chili powder
1 T. olive oil	1 can black beans, drained
½ c. peas	2 corn tortillas
	Hot sauce, to taste

1. Heat tofu and scallion in olive oil for 2–3 minutes,
   then add peas, corn, and chili powder. Cook another
   1–2 minutes, stirring frequently.
2. Reduce heat to medium low, and add black beans.
   Heat for 4–5 minutes, until well combined and
   heated through.
3. Place two corn tortillas in the bottom of a bowl, and
   spoon beans and tofu over the top. Season with hot
   sauce to taste.

Barley Vegetable Soup

*Barley and vegetable soup is an excellent "kitchen
sink" recipe, meaning that you can toss in just about
any fresh or frozen vegetables or spices you happen to
have on hand.* **Serves 6**

1 onion, chopped	1 (14-oz.) can crushed or diced tomatoes
2 carrots, sliced	½ t. parsley
2 ribs celery, chopped	½ t. thyme
2 T. olive oil	2 bay leaves
8 c. vegetable broth	Salt and pepper to taste
1 c. barley	
1½ c. frozen mixed vegetables	

1. In a large soup or stockpot, sauté the onion, carrots,
   and celery in olive oil for 3–5 minutes, just until
   onion is almost soft.
2. Reduce heat to medium low, and add remaining
   ingredients, except salt and pepper.
3. Bring to a simmer, cover, and allow to cook for at
   least 45 minutes, stirring occasionally.
4. Remove cover and allow to cook for 10 more minutes.
5. Remove bay leaves, season with salt and pepper to
   taste.

Glasses of Water Consumed: _____

Thoughts About Today: _____

_____

_____

What I Ate Today

Time	Food Item	Amount	Calories	Fat	Carbs	Fiber	Protein
TOTAL							

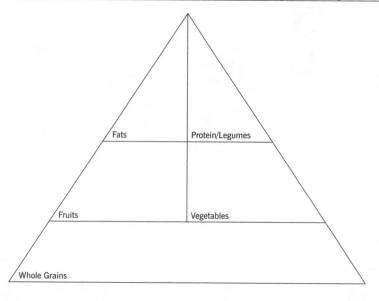

Breakfast

¾ c. frozen hash browns (about 250 calories) with ½ c. black beans, 1 oz. vegan cheese

Record nutritional values for your choice of frozen hash browns in today's journal. The nutritional values below are for black beans and vegan cheese only.

Cal.: 153.5; Fat: 2.45 g; Protein: 8.6 g; Sodium: 120.85 mg; Fiber: 7.5 g; Carbs.: 25.4 g; Sugar: 0 g; Zinc: 0.95 mg; Calcium: 223.2 mg; Iron: 1.8 mg; Vit. D: 0 mcg; Vit. B$_{12}$: 0 mcg

Lunch

1½ c. leftover Barley Vegetable Soup (see recipe in Week 10, Sat.), 1 slice whole grain toast, 1 small banana

Cal.: 468; Fat: 10.25 g; Protein: 14.35 g; Sodium: 315 mg; Fiber: 17.7 g; Carbs.: 83.9 g; Sugar: 15.57 g; Zinc: 2 mg; Calcium: 115.9 mg; Iron: 4.45 mg; Vit. D: 0 mcg; Vit. B$_{12}$: 0 mcg

Snack

2 Easy Banana Date Cookies, 1 small apple

Cal.: 283.5; Fat: 7.7 g; Protein: 1.92 g; Sodium: 6.9 mg; Fiber: 7.8 g; Carbs.: 58.6 g; Sugar: 37.5 g; Zinc: 0.54 mg; Calcium: 24.9 mg; Iron: 0.94 mg; Vit. D: 0 mcg; Vit. B$_{12}$: 0 mcg

Dinner

Saucy Kung Pao Tofu with ½ c. brown rice

Cal.: 517; Fat: 24.8 g; Protein: 27 g; Sodium: 526.8 mg; Fiber: 7.3 g; Carbs.: 53.6 g; Sugar: 1.54 g; Zinc: 3.8 mg; Calcium: 771.5 mg; Iron: 5.1 mg; Vit. D: 0 mcg; Vit. B$_{12}$: 0 mcg

Easy Banana Date Cookies

Yields 1 dozen

1 c. chopped, pitted dates	¼ t. vanilla
Water for soaking	1¾ c. coconut flakes
1 banana (medium ripe)	

1. Preheat oven to 375°F.
2. Cover dates in water, and soak for about 10 minutes until softened. Drain.
3. Process together the dates, banana, and vanilla until almost smooth.
4. Stir in coconut flakes by hand until thick. You may need a little more or less than 1¾ cups.
5. Drop by large tablespoonfuls onto ungreased cookie sheet, and bake 10–12 minutes or until done. Cookies will be soft and chewy.

Saucy Kung Pao Tofu

Serves 6

3 T. soy sauce	1 T. sesame oil
2 T. rice vinegar or cooking sherry	2 blocks firm or extra-firm tofu
1 red bell pepper, chopped	1 t. ginger powder
1 green bell pepper, chopped	½ c. water or vegetable broth
⅔ c. sliced mushrooms	½ t. sugar
3 cloves garlic	1½ t. cornstarch
3 small chili peppers, diced	2 green onions, chopped
1 t. red pepper flakes	½ c. peanuts
2 T. oil	

1. Whisk together the soy sauce, rice vinegar, and sesame oil in a shallow pan or zip-lock bag. Add tofu, and marinate for at least 1 hour; the longer, the better. Drain tofu, reserving marinade.
2. Sauté bell peppers, mushrooms, garlic, chili peppers, and red pepper flakes in oil for 2–3 minutes, then add tofu, and heat for another 1–2 minutes, until veggies are almost soft.
3. Reduce heat to medium low, and add marinade, ginger powder, water or vegetable broth, sugar, and cornstarch, whisking in the cornstarch to avoid lumps.
4. Heat a few more minutes, stirring constantly, until sauce has almost thickened.
5. Add green onions and peanuts, and heat for 1 more minute.

Glasses of Water Consumed: _____

Thoughts About Today: _____

_____

_____

What I Ate Today

Time	Food Item	Amount	Calories	Fat	Carbs	Fiber	Protein
TOTAL							

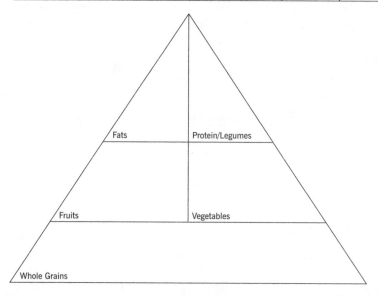

WEEK 10 IN REVIEW

I feel: _____
_____
_____
_____

My greatest food discovery this week was: _____
_____
_____
_____

This week's biggest vegan challenge was: _____
_____
_____
_____

New food I'd like to try: _____
_____
_____
_____

When I look back at this week, I most want to remember: _____
_____
_____
_____

Nutrition Totals

	Calories	Fat	Carbs	Fiber	Protein
Goal					
Actual					

WEEK 11

You're comfortable eating vegan, but have you considered veganizing the rest of your life? Start with the kitchen. Open up your cupboards and take a look. What's in your dish soap, laundry detergent, and kitchen cleaners? Are they full of chemicals? Tested on animals? Time to switch to something gentler on you, the animals, and Mother Earth. Make a note to pick up some natural cleaning products next time you run out. Next, take a look at the bathroom and the rest of your house. If your shampoos, cosmetics, and personal products are full of harsh chemicals, consider replacing them with organic, cruelty-free brands. Read the labels on your products. If it doesn't say "Not tested on animals" right there on the label, there's a very good chance it is. What a great excuse for a little retail therapy!

Treat yourself to one or two new animal- and earth-friendly personal products this week (you deserve it, of course!), and browse around for a few brands that you'd like to try in the future. If you're unsure where to start, the Internet is a great source for finding out which companies and brands do and don't test on animals.

Breakfast

1 c. whole grain cereal with ½ c. soy milk

Cal.: 178.33; Fat: 2.92 g; Protein: 6.17 g; Sodium: 267.83 mg; Fiber: 4.6 g; Carbs.: 33.43 g; Sugar: 7.17 g; Zinc: 20 mg; Calcium: 1373.33 mg; Iron: 24.7 mg; Vit. D: 54.7 mcg; Vit. B$_{12}$: 8.18 mcg

Lunch

Veggie burger with ¼ tomato, sliced, ¼ c. iceberg lettuce, mixed fruit salad with ½ apple, ½ banana, ½ c. strawberries, and ½ c. pineapple

Cal.: 466.83; Fat: 11.45 g; Protein: 20.88 g; Sodium: 628 mg; Fiber: 15.78 g; Carbs.: 75.85 g; Sugar: 31.6 g; Zinc: 2.35 mg; Calcium: 191.28 mg; Iron: 4.33 mg; Vit. D: 0 mcg; Vit. B$_{12}$: 1.4 mcg

Snack

1 Easy Banana Date Cookie (see recipe in Week 10, Sun.), 1 oz. almonds

Cal.: 264; Fat: 17.5 g; Protein: 6.66 g; Sodium: 3 mg; Fiber: 5.5 g; Carbs.: 25.1 g; Sugar: 12.1 g; Zinc: 1.12 mg; Calcium: 81.9 mg; Iron: 1.37 mg; Vit. D: 0 mcg; Vit. B$_{12}$: 0 mcg

Dinner

10 oz. Orange Ginger Mixed Veggie Stir-Fry with 1 c. rice noodles. 1 c. tomato juice (no salt added)

Cal.: 586; Fat: 8.4 g; Protein: 10.4 g; Sodium: 616.7 mg; Fiber: 8.6 g; Carbs.: 123.1 g; Sugar: 62.6 g; Zinc: 4.3 mg; Calcium: 166.3 mg; Iron: 4 mg; Vit. D: 0 mcg; Vit. B$_{12}$: 0 mcg

Orange Ginger Mixed Veggie Stir-Fry

Rice vinegar can be substituted for the apple cider vinegar, if you prefer. As with most stir-fry recipes, the vegetables are merely a suggestion; use your favorites or whatever looks like it's been sitting too long in your crisper. **Serves 4**

3 T. orange juice	2 T. oil
1 T. apple cider vinegar	1 bunch broccoli, chopped
2 T. soy sauce	½ c. sliced mushrooms
2 T. water	½ c. snap peas, chopped
1 T. maple syrup	1 carrot, sliced
1 t. powdered ginger	1 c. chopped cabbage or
2 cloves garlic, minced	bok choy

1. Whisk together the orange juice, vinegar, soy sauce, water, maple syrup, and powdered ginger.
2. Heat garlic in oil and add veggies. Allow to cook, stirring frequently, over high heat for 2–3 minutes, until just starting to get tender.
3. Add sauce and reduce heat. Simmer, stirring frequently, for another 3–4 minutes, or until veggies are cooked.

Cooking with Rice Noodles When stir-frying a saucy veggie dish, you can add quick-cooking Asian-style noodles right into the pan. Add some extra sauce ingredients and ¼ to ⅓ cup of water. Add the noodles, stir up the sauce, reduce the heat so the veggies don't scald, and keep covered for just a few minutes.

Monday

Glasses of Water Consumed: _____

Thoughts About Today: _____

_____

_____

What I Ate Today

Time	Food Item	Amount	Calories	Fat	Carbs	Fiber	Protein
TOTAL							

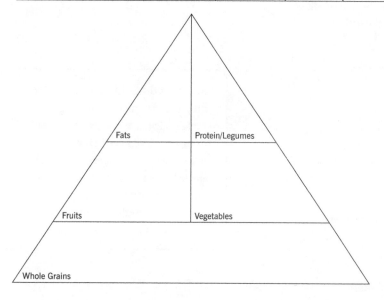

Tuesday

Breakfast

1 bagel with 2 T. almond butter

Cal.: 247; Fat: 10.4 g; Protein: 8.1 g; Sodium: 256.8 mg; Fiber: 1.9 g; Carbs.: 32.4 g; Sugar: 2.9 g; Zinc: 1.6 mg; Calcium: 93.9 mg; Iron: 4 mg; Vit. D: 0 mcg; Vit. B$_{12}$: 0 mcg

Lunch

10 oz. leftover Orange Ginger Mixed Veggie Stir-Fry (see recipe in Week 11, Mon.) with 1 c. rice noodles, 1 c. orange juice

Cal.: 655; Fat: 8.3 g; Protein: 10.6 g; Sodium: 592.4 mg; Fiber: 7.6 g; Carbs.: 138.8 g; Sugar: 76 g; Zinc: 3.9 mg; Calcium: 492 mg; Iron: 5.25 mg; Vit. D: 0 mcg; Vit. B$_{12}$: 0.41 mcg

Snack

Mixed veggies (½ cucumber, 2 oz. baby carrots, ½ c. broccoli) with 2 T. hummus

Cal.: 116.92; Fat: 3.32 g; Protein: 5.38 g; Sodium: 189.5 mg; Fiber: 6.52 g; Carbs.: 19.37 g; Sugar: 6.12 g; Zinc: 1.27 mg; Calcium: 81.63 mg; Iron: 2.18 mg; Vit. D: 0 mcg; Vit. B$_{12}$: 0 mcg

Dinner

8 oz. Mexican Rice with Corn and Peppers, ½ c. black beans, side green salad with 2 c. romaine lettuce, 1 tomato, and 1 diced cucumber, 2 T. Goddess Dressing (see recipe in Week 1, Mon.)

Cal.: 526.2; Fat: 21.6 g; Protein: 14.5 g; Sodium: 521.2 mg; Fiber: 14.32 g; Carbs.: 78.9 g; Sugar: 18.36 g; Zinc: 3.08 mg; Calcium: 190.5 mg; Iron: 7.32 mg; Vit. D: 0 mcg; Vit. B$_{12}$: 0 mcg

Mexican Rice with Corn and Peppers

Although Mexican rice is usually just a filling for burritos or served as a side dish, this recipe loads up the veggies, making it hearty enough for a main dish. Use frozen or canned veggies if you need to save time.

Serves 4

2 cloves garlic, minced	Kernels from one ear of corn
1 c. rice	1 carrot, diced
2 T. olive oil	1 t. chili powder
3 c. vegetable broth	½ t. cumin
1 c. tomato paste (or 4 large tomatoes, pureed)	⅓ t. oregano
1 green bell pepper, chopped	⅓ t. cayenne pepper (or to taste)
1 red bell pepper, chopped	⅓ t. salt

1. Add garlic, rice, and olive oil to a large skillet and heat on medium-high heat, stirring frequently. Toast the rice until just golden brown, about 2–3 minutes.
2. Reduce heat and add vegetable broth and remaining ingredients.
3. Bring to a simmer, cover, and allow to cook until liquid is absorbed and rice is cooked, about 20–25 minutes, stirring occasionally.
4. Adjust seasonings to taste.

Concerned about Calcium? Yes, you do need to make sure you get enough calcium as a vegan, but to build strong bones, you need exercise as well as calcium, so vegan or not, diet is only half the equation. Reliable vegan sources of calcium include spinach, kale, soy milk, fortified orange juice, tahini, and tofu.

Glasses of Water Consumed: _____

Thoughts About Today: _____

_____

_____

What I Ate Today

Time	Food Item	Amount	Calories	Fat	Carbs	Fiber	Protein
TOTAL							

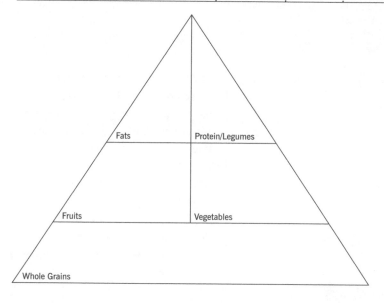

Fats | Protein/Legumes

Fruits | Vegetables

Whole Grains

Wednesday

Breakfast

1 vegan sausage patty on an English muffin with 1 (1-oz.) slice vegan cheese, 1 small apple

Cal.: 337.5; Fat: 6.4 g; Protein: 16.8 g; Sodium: 629.5 mg; Fiber: 6.1 g; Carbs.: 56 g; Sugar: 18.3 g; Zinc: 0.8 mg; Calcium: 313.9 mg; Iron: 4.04 mg; Vit. D: 0 mcg; Vit. B$_{12}$: 2.1 mcg

Lunch

8 oz. leftover Mexican Rice with Corn and Peppers (see recipe in Week 11, Tues.) in a taco shell with 1 oz. vegan cheese, 1 tomato, sliced, ¼ c. iceberg lettuce, 1 c. strawberries

Cal.: 162.43; Fat: 5.25 g; Protein: 3.775 g; Sodium: 171.65 mg; Fiber: 4.88 g; Carbs.: 28.1 g; Sugar: 9.8 g; Zinc: 0.55 mg; Calcium: 249.9 mg; Iron: 1.1 mg; Vit. D: 0 mcg; Vit. B$_{12}$: 0 mcg

Snack

1 oz. almonds with 1 oz. cranberries, 1 small apple

Cal.: 201.1; Fat: 7.4 g; Protein: 3.35 g; Sodium: 2.05 mg; Fiber: 18.2 g; Carbs.: 35.2 g; Sugar: 25.15 g; Zinc: 0.55 mg; Calcium: 47.25 mg; Iron: 0.75 mg; Vit. D: 0 mcg; Vit. B$_{12}$: 0 mcg

Dinner

1½ c. Black Bean and Butternut Squash Chili (see recipe in Week 1, Wed.), side green salad with 2 c. romaine lettuce, 1 tomato, and 1 diced cucumber, 2 T. Goddess Dressing (see recipe in Week 1, Mon.)

Cal.: 733.2; Fat: 19.1 g; Protein: 35.5 g; Sodium: 722.2 mg; Fiber: 27.12 g; Carbs.: 112.9 g; Sugar: 18.76 g; Zinc: 6.58 mg; Calcium: 350.5 mg; Iron: 10.32 mg; Vit. D: 0 mcg; Vit. B$_{12}$: 0 mcg

Craving Haggis? It's probably not haggis you're going to miss when going vegan, but if it is, there's a vegan substitute! Besides the more common mock chicken and beef products, some of the unbelievable vegan substitutes on the market today include black pudding, vegan caviar, prawns, mutton, and even vegetarian squid and eel.

Glasses of Water Consumed: _____

Thoughts About Today: _____

_____

_____

What I Ate Today

Time	Food Item	Amount	Calories	Fat	Carbs	Fiber	Protein
TOTAL							

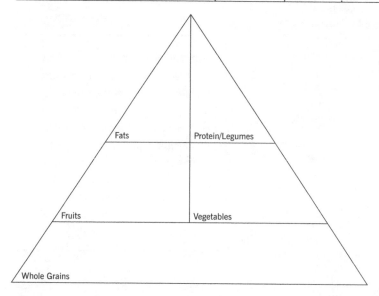

Thursday

Breakfast

1 c. Cream of Wheat, 1 small banana, 1 c. soy hot chocolate

Cal.: 321.4; Fat: 4.9 g; Protein: 17.5 g; Sodium: 555 mg; Fiber: 6 g; Carbs.: 94.6 g; Sugar: 42.6 g; Zinc: 1.92 mg; Calcium: 759.1 mg; Iron: 14.46 mg; Vit. D: 2.7 mcg; Vit. B_{12}: 3 mcg

Lunch

1½ c. leftover Black Bean and Butternut Squash Chili (see recipe in Week 1, Wed.), 1 c. pineapple

Cal.: 612.5; Fat: 7 g; Protein: 29.9 g; Sodium: 497.7 mg; Fiber: 23.3 g; Carbs.: 112.6 g; Sugar: 25.3 g; Zinc: 5.2 mg; Calcium: 228.5 mg; Iron: 7.5 mg; Vit. D: 0 mcg; Vit. B_{12}: 0 mcg

Snack

Mixed veggies (½ cucumber, 2 oz. baby carrots, ½ c. broccoli) with 2 T. Goddess Dressing (see recipe in Week 1, Mon.)

Cal.: 186.92; Fat: 12.12 g; Protein: 5.18 g; Sodium: 97.9 mg; Fiber: 5.84 g; Carbs.: 18.37 g; Sugar: 6.48 g; Zinc: 1.25 mg; Calcium: 122.23 mg; Iron: 2.6 mg; Vit. D: 0 mcg; Vit. B_{12}: 0 mcg

Dinner

10 oz. Savory Stuffed Acorn Squash

Cal.: 206; Fat: 12 g; Protein: 4.3 g; Sodium: 567 mg; Fiber: 5.5 g; Carbs.: 24 g; Sugar: 0.77 g; Zinc: 0 mg; Calcium: 91 mg; Iron: 2.6 mg; Vit. D: 0 mcg; Vit. B_{12}: 0 mcg

Savory Stuffed Acorn Squash

All the flavors of fall baked into one nutritious dish. Use fresh herbs, if you have them, and breathe in deep to savor the impossibly magical aromas coming from your kitchen. **Serves 4**

2 acorn squash
1 t. garlic powder
½ t. salt
2 ribs celery, chopped
1 onion, diced
½ c. sliced mushrooms
2 T. vegan margarine or oil

¼ c. chopped walnuts
1 T. soy sauce
1 t. parsley
½ t. thyme
½ t. sage
Salt and pepper, to taste
½ c. grated vegan cheese (optional)

1. Preheat oven to 350°F. Chop the squash in half and scrape out any stringy bits and seeds.
2. Sprinkle squash with garlic powder and salt, then place cut-side down on a baking sheet and bake for 30 minutes or until almost soft, then remove from oven.
3. In a large skillet, heat celery, onion, and mushrooms in vegan margarine until soft, about 4–5 minutes.
4. Add walnuts, soy sauce, parsley, thyme, and sage, stirring to combine well, and season generously with salt and pepper. Heat for another 1–2 minutes, until fragrant.
5. Fill squash with mushroom mixture and sprinkle with optional vegan cheese. Bake another 5–10 minutes, until squash is soft.

Did You Know? Religious ascetics and philosophers have dabbled with vegetarian and mostly vegan diets throughout history. Among the ancient Greeks, mathematician and philosopher Pythagoras mentored a group of vegetarians in the sixth century B.C., and at the same time in India, the ancient Jains were already practicing ahimsa, pledging not to kill by avoiding animal flesh and eggs.

Thursday

Glasses of Water Consumed: _____

Thoughts About Today: _____

_____

_____

What I Ate Today

Time	Food Item	Amount	Calories	Fat	Carbs	Fiber	Protein
TOTAL							

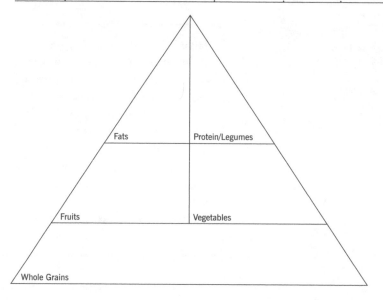

Friday

Breakfast

1 Strawberry Protein Smoothie, 1 small banana

Cal.: 293.9; **Fat:** 5.8 g; **Protein:** 11.1 g; **Sodium:** 14 mg; **Fiber:** 5.9 g; **Carbs.:** 57.1 g; **Sugar:** 32.4 g; **Zinc:** 1.5 mg; **Calcium:** 167.1 mg; **Iron:** 2.1 mg; **Vit. D:** 0 mcg; **Vit. B$_{12}$:** 0 mcg

Lunch

Caesar salad with 2 c. romaine lettuce, 6 oz. vegetarian chicken, and 1 T. Goddess Dressing (see recipe in Week 1, Mon.), 1 small apple, 1 c. orange juice

Cal.: 495.5; **Fat:** 16.2 g; **Protein:** 22.1 g; **Sodium:** 225.3 mg; **Fiber:** 13.16 g; **Carbs.:** 71.7 g; **Sugar:** 38.28 g; **Zinc:** 0.49 mg; **Calcium:** 470.4 mg; **Iron:** 33.56 mg; **Vit. D:** 0 mcg; **Vit. B$_{12}$:** 0.41 mcg

Snack

Mixed fruit salad with ½ apple, ½ banana, ½ c. strawberries, and ½ c. pineapple

Cal.: 149.25; **Fat:** 0.65 g; **Protein:** 1.7 g; **Sodium:** 2.85 mg; **Fiber:** 5.75 g; **Carbs.:** 38.5 g; **Sugar:** 25.8 g; **Zinc:** 0.35 mg; **Calcium:** 29.9 mg; **Iron:** 0.8 mg; **Vit. D:** 0 mcg; **Vit. B$_{12}$:** 0 mcg

Dinner

5 oz. Garlic Miso and Onion Soup with 1 c. soba noodles, 1 c. steamed spinach with 16 g nutritional yeast

Cal.: 372.4; **Fat:** 7.4 g; **Protein:** 29.1 g; **Sodium:** 1984.4 mg; **Fiber:** 11.7 g; **Carbs.:** 57.1 g; **Sugar:** 7 g; **Zinc:** 6.6 mg; **Calcium:** 302.6 mg; **Iron:** 9.5 mg; **Vit. D:** 0 mcg; **Vit. B$_{12}$:** 7.8 mcg

Garlic Miso and Onion Soup

Serves 2

4 c. water or vegetable broth

½ c. sliced shiitake mushrooms

3 scallions, chopped

½ onion, chopped

4 cloves garlic, minced

¾ t. garlic powder

2 T. soy sauce

1 t. sesame oil

1 block silken tofu, diced

⅓ c. miso

1 T. chopped seaweed, any kind (optional)

1. Combine all ingredients except for miso and seaweed in a large soup or stockpot and bring to a slow simmer. Cook, uncovered, for 10–12 minutes.
2. Reduce heat and stir in miso and seaweed, being careful not to boil.
3. Heat, stirring to dissolve miso, for another 5 minutes, until onions and mushrooms are soft.

Miso Trivia Miso is available in a variety of interchangeable flavors and colors, red, white, and barley miso being the most common. It's really a personal preference which type you use. Asian grocers stock miso at about a third of the price of natural-food stores, so if you're lucky enough to have one in your neighborhood, it's worth a trip. Boiling miso destroys some of its beneficial enzymes, so when making soup, be sure to heat it to just below a simmer.

Glasses of Water Consumed: _____

Thoughts About Today: _____

_____

_____

What I Ate Today

Time	Food Item	Amount	Calories	Fat	Carbs	Fiber	Protein
TOTAL							

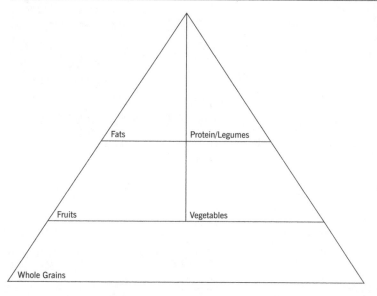

Fats

Protein/Legumes

Fruits

Vegetables

Whole Grains

Breakfast

6 oz. Rosemary Tempeh Hash, 1 c. chocolate soy milk

Cal.: 399; **Fat:** 15.5 g; **Protein:** 18 g; **Sodium:** 153 mg; **Fiber:** 5.5 g; **Carbs.:** 50 g; **Sugar:** 16 g; **Zinc:** 1.17 mg; **Calcium:** 373 mg; **Iron:** 4.38 mg; **Vit. D:** 0 mcg; **Vit. B$_{12}$:** 3 mcg

Lunch

6 oz. Macro-Inspired Veggie Bowl

Cal.: 453; **Fat:** 31 g; **Protein:** 17 g; **Sodium:** 408 mg; **Fiber:** 7.4 g; **Carbs.:** 21 g; **Sugar:** 1.7 g; **Zinc:** 1.8 mg; **Calcium:** 409 mg; **Iron:** 7.3 mg; **Vit. D:** 0 mcg; **Vit. B$_{12}$:** 0 mcg

Snack

200 calories of whole grain chips with ¼ c. Black Bean Guacamole (see recipe in Week 2, Tues.)

Record nutritional values for your choice of whole grain chips in today's journal. The nutritional values below are for the guacamole only.

Cal.: 91; **Fat:** 8.4 g; **Protein:** 1.1 g; **Sodium:** 86 mg; **Fiber:** 3.8 g; **Carbs.:** 4.9 g; **Sugar:** 0.4 g; **Zinc:** 0 mg; **Calcium:** 10 mg; **Iron:** 0.36 mg; **Vit. D:** 0 mcg; **Vit. B$_{12}$:** 0 mcg

Dinner

6 oz. Easy Three Bean Casserole, side green salad with 2 c. romaine lettuce, 1 tomato, and 1 diced cucumber, 2 T. Goddess Dressing (see recipe in Week 1, Mon.)

Cal.: 604.2; **Fat:** 13.6 g; **Protein:** 30.5 g; **Sodium:** 554.2 mg; **Fiber:** 26.12 g; **Carbs.:** 99.9 g; **Sugar:** 27.76 g; **Zinc:** 5.88 mg; **Calcium:** 291.5 mg; **Iron:** 9.92 mg; **Vit. D:** 0.79 mcg; **Vit. B$_{12}$:** 0 mcg

Rosemary Tempeh Hash

Serves 4

2 potatoes, diced
Water for boiling
1 (8-oz.) package tempeh, cubed
2 T. olive oil
2 green onions, chopped
1 t. chili powder
1 t. rosemary
Salt and pepper to taste

1. Cover the potatoes with water in a large pot and bring to a boil. Cook just until potatoes are almost soft, about 15 minutes. Drain.
2. In a large pan, sauté the potatoes and tempeh in olive oil for 3–4 minutes, lightly browning tempeh on all sides.
3. Add green onions, chili powder, and rosemary, stirring to combine, and heat for 3–4 more minutes. Season well with salt and pepper.

Macro-Inspired Veggie Bowl

Serves 8

2 c. cooked brown rice
1 block baked tofu, chopped into cubes
1 head broccoli, steamed and chopped
1 red or yellow bell pepper, sliced thin
1 c. bean sprouts
1 c. Goddess Dressing
½ c. pumpkin seeds

1. Divide brown rice into four bowls.
2. Top each bowl with tofu, broccoli, bell pepper, and bean sprouts.
3. Drizzle with dressing and pumpkin seeds.

Easy Three Bean Casserole

Serves 8

1 15 oz. can vegetarian baked beans
1 15 oz. can black beans, drained
1 15 oz. can kidney beans, drained
1 onion, chopped
⅓ c. ketchup
3 T. apple cider vinegar
⅓ c. brown sugar
2 t. mustard powder
2 t. garlic powder
4 vegan hot dogs, cooked and chopped (optional)

1. Pre-heat oven to 350°F.
2. Combine all ingredients, except vegan hot dogs, in a large casserole dish.
3. Bake for 55 minutes, uncovered. Add precooked vegan hot dogs just before serving.

Glasses of Water Consumed: _____

Thoughts About Today: _____

_____

_____

What I Ate Today

Time	Food Item	Amount	Calories	Fat	Carbs	Fiber	Protein
TOTAL							

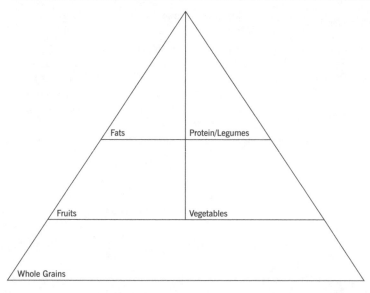

Sunday

Breakfast

2 oz. polenta with ½ c. black beans, 2 slices (1 oz.) vegan cheese

Cal.: 355.5; Fat: 4.45 g; Protein: 13.2 g; Sodium: 140.45 mg; Fiber: 11.5 g; Carbs.: 68.4 g; Sugar: 0.4 g; Zinc: 1.95 mg; Calcium: 226.6 mg; Iron: 3.8 mg; Vit. D: 0 mcg; Vit. B$_{12}$: 0 mcg

Lunch

¾ c. Five-Minute Vegan Pasta Salad, 1 small banana

Cal.: 454.9; Fat: 17.3 g; Protein: 8.8 g; Sodium: 860 mg; Fiber: 5.6 g; Carbs.: 73.1 g; Sugar: 18.4 g; Zinc: 0.2 mg; Calcium: 22.1 mg; Iron: 2.9 mg; Vit. D: 0 mcg; Vit. B$_{12}$: 0 mcg

Snack

1 oz. dried apricots, 1 oz. dried cranberries

Cal.: 153.7; Fat: 0.5 g; Protein: 0.9 g; Sodium: 3.6 mg; Fiber: 3.6 g; Carbs.: 40.6 g; Sugar: 33.2 g; Zinc: 0.1 mg; Calcium: 18.2 mg; Iron: 0.8 mg; Vit. D: 0 mcg; Vit. B$_{12}$: 0 mcg

Dinner

5.5 oz. Tofu "Fish" Sticks, 1 steamed sweet potato, 1 ear corn on the cob with 16 g nutritional yeast

Cal.: 595; Fat: 13.8 g; Protein: 33.7 g; Sodium: 320 mg; Fiber: 10.1 g; Carbs.: 94.3 g; Sugar: 7.3 g; Zinc: 6.3 mg; Calcium: 684.2 mg; Iron: 7.4 mg; Vit. D: 0 mcg; Vit. B$_{12}$: 0 mcg

---

Five-Minute Vegan Pasta Salad

Once you've got the pasta cooked and cooled, this takes just 5 minutes to assemble, as it's made with store-bought dressing. A balsamic vinaigrette or tomato dressing would also work well. **Serves 4**

4 c. cooked pasta	1 tomato, chopped
¾ c. vegan Italian salad dressing	1 avocado, diced (optional)
3 scallions, chopped	Salt and pepper to taste
½ c. sliced black olives	

Toss together all ingredients. Allow to chill for at least 1½ hours before serving, if time allows, to allow flavors to combine.

Tofu "Fish" Sticks

Adding seaweed and lemon juice to baked and breaded tofu gives it a "fishy" taste. Crumbled nori sushi sheets would work well, too, if you can't find kelp or dulse flakes. You could also pan-fry these "fish" sticks in a bit of oil instead of baking, if you prefer. **Serves 4**

½ c. flour	1 T. Old Bay seasoning blend
⅓ c. soy milk	1 t. onion powder
2 T. lemon juice	1 block extra-firm tofu, well pressed
1½ c. fine ground bread crumbs	
2 T. kelp or dulse seaweed flakes	

1. Preheat oven to 350°F.
2. Place flour in a shallow bowl or pie tin and set aside. Combine the soy milk and lemon juice in a separate shallow bowl or pie tin. In a third bowl or pie tin, combine the bread crumbs, kelp, Old Bay, and onion powder.
3. Slice tofu into 12½-inch-thick strips. Place each strip into the flour mixture to coat well, then dip into the soy milk. Next, place each strip into the bread crumbs, gently patting to coat well.
4. Bake for 15–20 minutes, turn once, then bake for another 10–15 minutes, or until crispy.

Date ____ / ____ / ____

Glasses of Water Consumed: _____

Thoughts About Today: _____

_____

_____

What I Ate Today

Time	Food Item	Amount	Calories	Fat	Carbs	Fiber	Protein
TOTAL							

Fats

Protein/Legumes

Fruits

Vegetables

Whole Grains

Instant Additions Open up a jar and instantly add color, flavor, and texture to a basic pasta salad. What's in your cupboard? Try capers, roasted red peppers, canned veggies, jarred pimentos, sun-dried tomatoes, or even mandarin oranges or sliced beets. Snip in any leftover fresh herbs you have on hand.

WEEK 11 IN REVIEW

I feel: _____
_____
_____
_____
_____

My greatest food discovery this week was: _____
_____
_____
_____
_____

This week's biggest vegan challenge was: _____
_____
_____
_____
_____

New food I'd like to try: _____
_____
_____
_____
_____

When I look back at this week, I most want to remember: _____
_____
_____
_____
_____

Nutrition Totals

	Calories	Fat	Carbs	Fiber	Protein
Goal					
Actual					

WEEK 12

Being vegan is about so much more than just eating a healthy diet. It's about choosing to live a healthy and compassionate lifestyle; it's about sleeping better at night, knowing your actions are in line with your ethical values; and it's about celebrating all of the life-giving foods that Mother Nature has to offer. This weekend, you will have been vegan for twelve weeks! It's time to celebrate! A few ideas? Cook up your favorite meal, and enjoy it with a lovely bottle of wine. Or venture out and try everything on the menu at the local vegan restaurant. Special-order a vegan cake, and share it with friends.

But before you do, make sure you're well prepared to continue eating vegan and healthy from here on out on your own. Do you have a plan for week thirteen? By now, you should be so comfortable eating vegan that you don't need one. You have plenty of breakfast, lunch, and dinner ideas in your regular repertoire of foods to choose from. If you're still uncertain about getting in all your nutrients, try mixing and matching a few of the meals throughout this book.

Final words of wisdom? Enjoy a bit of vegan chocolate and vegan ice cream from time to time, and don't forget to get your B_{12}! Welcome to the wonderful world of veganism! Doesn't it feel fantastic?

Breakfast

1 T. peanut butter with 1 T. sugar-free jam on 2 slices whole grain bread, 1 small banana

Cal.: 370; Fat: 10.5 g; Protein: 10.5 g; Sodium: 228 mg; Fiber: 7.4 g; Carbs.: 58.7 g; Sugar: 24.4 g; Zinc: 1 mg; Calcium: 58.3 mg; Iron: 1.7 mg; Vit. D: 0 mcg; Vit. B_{12}: 0 mcg

Snack

Mixed veggies (½ cucumber, 2 oz. baby carrots, ½ c. broccoli) with 2 T. hummus, 1 oz. cashews

Cal.: 271.92; Fat: 15.62 g; Protein: 10.48 g; Sodium: 192.9 mg; Fiber: 7.42 g; Carbs.: 28.57 g; Sugar: 7.82 g; Zinc: 2.87 mg; Calcium: 92.03 mg; Iron: 4.08 mg; Vit. D: 0 mcg; Vit. B_{12}: 0 mcg

Lunch

Burrito with 1 flour tortilla, ½ c. beef substitute, ½ tomato, and ½ c. iceberg lettuce, 1 c. tomato juice (no salt added)

Cal.: 428.1; Fat: 5.6 g; Protein: 24.65 g; Sodium: 977 mg; Fiber: 14 g; Carbs.: 65.85 g; Sugar: 15.9 g; Zinc: 2.25 mg; Calcium: 128.95 mg; Iron: 4.9 mg; Vit. D: 0 mcg; Vit. B_{12}: 0 mcg

Dinner

6 oz. Greek Lemon Rice with Spinach and 4½ oz. Lemon Basil Tofu

Cal.: 402; Fat: 23.3 g; Protein: 22.7 g; Sodium: 559 mg; Fiber: 6.2 g; Carbs.: 29.7 g; Sugar: 6.93 g; Zinc: 3.17 mg; Calcium: 800 mg; Iron: 6.6 mg; Vit. D: mcg; Vit. B_{12}: mcg

Greek Lemon Rice with Spinach

Greek spanakorizo is seasoned with fresh lemon, herbs, and black pepper. **Serves 4**

1 onion, chopped	2 T. chopped fresh parsley
4 cloves garlic, minced	1 T. chopped fresh mint or dill (optional)
2 T. olive oil	
¾ c. rice	2 T. lemon juice
2½ c. water or vegetable broth	½ t. salt
1 (8-oz.) can tomato paste	½ t. fresh ground black pepper
2 bunches fresh spinach, trimmed	

1. Sauté onions and garlic in olive oil for just 1–2 minutes, then add rice, stirring to lightly toast.
2. Add water or vegetable broth, cover, and heat for 10–12 minutes.
3. Add tomato paste, spinach, and parsley. Cover, and cook for another 5 minutes or until spinach is wilted and rice is cooked.
4. Stir in fresh mint or dill, lemon juice, salt, and pepper.

Lemon Basil Tofu

Moist and chewy, this zesty baked tofu is reminiscent of lemon chicken. Serve drizzled with extra marinade, or use the extra marinade as a salad dressing. **Serves 6**

3 T. lemon juice	3 T. olive oil
1 T. soy sauce	2 T. chopped basil, plus extra for garnish
2 t. apple cider vinegar	
1 T. Dijon mustard	2 blocks firm or extra-firm tofu, well pressed
¾ t. sugar	

1. Whisk together all ingredients, except tofu, and transfer to a baking dish or casserole pan.
2. Slice the tofu into ½-inch-thick strips or triangles.
3. Place the tofu in the marinade and coat well. Allow to marinate for at least 1 hour or overnight, being sure tofu is well coated in marinade.
4. Preheat oven to 350°F.
5. Bake for 15 minutes, turn over, then bake for another 10–12 minutes or until done. Garnish with a few extra bits of chopped fresh basil.

Date _____ / _____ / _____

Glasses of Water Consumed: _____

Thoughts About Today: _____

_____

_____

What I Ate Today

Time	Food Item	Amount	Calories	Fat	Carbs	Fiber	Protein
TOTAL							

A High-Protein Rice? Wild rice is not actually rice, but rather a seed. With almost 7 grams of protein per cup when cooked, wild rice can be an excellent source of protein. Add ¼ cup wild rice per cup of white rice to any recipe that calls for regular white rice for an extra protein boost.

Tuesday

Breakfast

1 c. instant grits with 1 (1-oz.) slice vegan cheese, 1 c. applesauce

Cal.: 285; Fat: 2.7 g; Protein: 4.8 g; Sodium: 664.9 mg; Fiber: 3.4 g; Carbs.: 63.6 g; Sugar: 23.1 g; Zinc: 0.3 mg; Calcium: 217.1 mg; Iron: 2.1 mg; Vit. D: 0 mcg; Vit. B$_{12}$: 0 mcg

Lunch

4½ oz. leftover Greek Lemon Rice with Spinach and Lemon Basil Tofu (see recipes in Week 12, Mon.), 1 small apple

Cal.: 258.5; Fat: 7.6 g; Protein: 5.1 g; Sodium: 376.5 mg; Fiber: 7.6 g; Carbs.: 45.6 g; Sugar: 22.2 g; Zinc: 1.07 mg; Calcium: 73.9 mg; Iron: 3.4 mg; Vit. D: 0 mcg; Vit. B$_{12}$: 0 mcg

Snack

1 c. popcorn with 8 g nutritional yeast

Cal.: 53.1; Fat: 0.55 g; Protein: 5 g; Sodium: 2.8 mg; Fiber: 3.2 g; Carbs.: 8.7 g; Sugar: 0.5 g; Zinc: 1.8 mg; Calcium: 0.8 mg; Iron: 0.55 mg; Vit. D: 0 mcg; Vit. B$_{12}$: 3.9 mcg

Dinner

12 oz. Fiery Basil and Eggplant Stir-Fry with 1 c. rice noodles

Cal.: 448; Fat: 19.4 g; Protein: 22.6 g; Sodium: 718.4 mg; Fiber: 9.4 g; Carbs.: 61.8 g; Sugar: 3.5 g; Zinc: 2.7 mg; Calcium: 767 mg; Iron: 4.2 mg; Vit. D: 0 mcg; Vit. B$_{12}$: 0 mcg

Fiery Basil and Eggplant Stir-Fry

Holy basil, called tulsi, *is revered in Vishnu temples across India and is frequently used in Ayurvedic healing. It lends a fantastically spicy flavor, but regular basil will also do.* **Serves 3**

3 cloves garlic, minced	1 red bell pepper, chopped
3 small fresh chili peppers, minced	⅓ c. sliced mushrooms
1 block firm or extra-firm tofu, pressed and diced	3 T. water
	2 T. soy sauce
2 T. olive oil	1 t. lemon juice
1 eggplant, chopped	⅓ c. fresh Thai basil or holy basil

1. Sauté the garlic, chili peppers, and tofu in olive oil for 4–6 minutes until tofu is lightly golden.
2. Add eggplant, bell pepper, mushrooms, water, and soy sauce, and heat, stirring frequently, for 5–6 minutes or until eggplant is almost soft.
3. Add lemon juice and basil, and cook for another 1–2 minutes, just until basil is wilted.

Glasses of Water Consumed: _____

Thoughts About Today: _____

_____

_____

What I Ate Today

Time	Food Item	Amount	Calories	Fat	Carbs	Fiber	Protein
TOTAL							

Fats

Protein/Legumes

Fruits

Vegetables

Whole Grains

Types of Basil Sweet Italian basil may be the most common, but other varieties can add a layer of sensually enticing flavor. Lemon basil is identifiable by its lighter green color and fresh citrusy scent. For tonight's dinner, look for spicy holy basil or Thai basil with a purplish stem and jagged leaf edge for a delightfully scorching flavor.

Wednesday

Breakfast

1 c. whole grain cereal with ½ c. soy milk

Cal.: 178.33; Fat: 2.92 g; Protein: 6.17 g; Sodium: 267.83 mg; Fiber: 4.6 g; Carbs.: 33.43 g; Sugar: 7.17 g; Zinc: 20 mg; Calcium: 1373.33 mg; Iron: 24.7 mg; Vit. D: 54.7 mcg; Vit. B$_{12}$: 8.18 mcg

Lunch

Grilled cheese sandwich with 2 slices whole grain bread, 2 (1-oz.) slices vegan cheese, 200 calories of tomato soup, 1 small banana

Record nutritional values for your choice of tomato soup in today's journal. The nutritional values below are for the grilled cheese sandwich only.

Cal.: 295; Fat: 6.5 g; Protein: 9.4 g; Sodium: 461.5 mg; Fiber: 7.4 g; Carbs.: 53.2 g; Sugar: 18.9 g; Zinc: 0.9 mg; Calcium: 462.1 mg; Iron: 1.6 mg; Vit. D: 0 mcg; Vit. B$_{12}$: 0 mcg

Snack

200 calories of whole grain crackers with 3 T. olive tapenade

Record nutritional values for your choice of whole grain crackers in today's journal. The nutritional values below are for the olive tapenade only.

Cal.: 90; Fat: 6 g; Protein: 0 g; Sodium: 480 mg; Fiber: 0 g; Carbs.: 3 g; Sugar: 0 g; Zinc: 0 mg; Calcium: 69 mg; Iron: 2.1 mg; Vit. D: 0 mcg; Vit. B$_{12}$: 0 mcg

Dinner

1 c. Indian Curried Lentil Soup with 1 c. quinoa

Cal.: 467; Fat: 10 g; Protein: 21.1 g; Sodium: 687 mg; Fiber: 21.2 g; Carbs.: 71.4 g; Sugar: 2.6 g; Zinc: 4.4 mg; Calcium: 72.5 mg; Iron: 6.6 mg; Vit. D: 0 mcg; Vit. B$_{12}$: 0 mcg

Indian Curried Lentil Soup

Similar to a traditional Indian lentil dal recipe but with added vegetables to make it into an entrée, this lentil soup is perfect as is or perhaps paired with rice or some warmed Indian flatbread. **Serves 4**

1 onion, diced	1 c. yellow or green lentils
1 carrot, sliced	2¾ c. vegetable broth
3 whole cloves	2 large tomatoes, chopped
2 T. vegan margarine	1 t. salt
1 t. cumin	¼ t. black pepper
1 t. turmeric	1 t. lemon juice

1. In a large soup or stockpot, sauté the onion, carrot, and cloves in margarine until onions are just turning soft, about 3 minutes. Add cumin and turmeric and toast for 1 minute, stirring constantly to avoid burning.
2. Reduce heat to medium low and add lentils, vegetable broth, tomatoes, and salt. Bring to a simmer, cover, and cook for 35–40 minutes, or until lentils are done.
3. Season with black pepper and lemon juice just before serving.

Time-Saving Simmer Sauces If you like ethnic food but don't like spending time in the kitchen, an array of vegan simmer sauces is at your fingertips. From Thai curry and satay sauces to Indian masalas, these simmer sauces can be mixed with tofu, veggies, and a grain for a quick and easy meal. These are usually found in the ethnic foods aisle, but you might also find some near the salad dressings and barbecue sauces.

Date ____ / ____ / ____

Glasses of Water Consumed: _____

Thoughts About Today: _____

_____

_____

What I Ate Today

Time	Food Item	Amount	Calories	Fat	Carbs	Fiber	Protein
TOTAL							

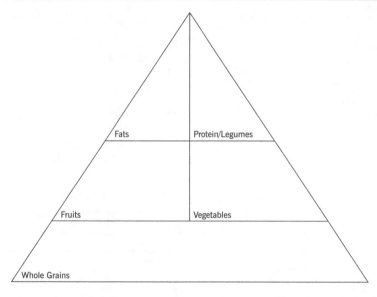

Fats

Protein/Legumes

Fruits

Vegetables

Whole Grains

Thursday

Breakfast

1 English muffin with 1 vegetarian sausage patty, ¼ medium tomato, sliced, and 2 oz. avocado slices

Cal.: 315.13; Fat: 12.35 g; Protein: 16.88 g; Sodium: 513.55 mg; Fiber: 6.88 g; Carbs.: 36.4 g; Sugar: 4 g; Zinc: 1.15 mg; Calcium: 114.88 mg; Iron: 4.32 mg; Vit. D: 0 mcg; Vit. B_{12}: 2.1 mcg

Lunch

1 c. leftover Indian Curried Lentil Soup (see recipe in Week 12, Wed.) with 1 slice whole grain toast

Cal.: 314.1; Fat: 7.5 g; Protein: 16.5 g; Sodium: 784 mg; Fiber: 17.9 g; Carbs.: 43.3 g; Sugar: 4.3 g; Zinc: 2.8 mg; Calcium: 67.6 mg; Iron: 4.5 mg; Vit. D: 0 mcg; Vit. B_{12}: 0 mcg

Snack

1 medium apple with ½ T. peanut butter and ½ oz. raisins, 1 oz. almonds

Cal.: 330.35; Fat: 18.15 g; Protein: 9.25 g; Sodium: 4.85 mg; Fiber: 8 g; Carbs.: 39.3g; Sugar: 25.4 g; Zinc: 1.05 mg; Calcium: 89.8 mg; Iron: 1.45 mg; Vit. D: 0 mcg; Vit. B_{12}: 0 mcg

Dinner

7 oz. Creamy Sun-Dried Tomato Pasta, Greek spinach salad with 2 c. fresh spinach, ½ red bell pepper, 2 T. black olives, ¼ c. chopped artichoke hearts, and 2 T. Goddess Dressing (see recipe in Week 1, Mon.)

Cal.: 788; Fat: 35.9 g; Protein: 33.6 g; Sodium: 1268 mg; Fiber: 12.84 g; Carbs.: 96.4 g; Sugar: 12.52 g; Zinc: 3.06 mg; Calcium: 767 mg; Iron: 13.54 mg; Vit. D: 0 mcg; Vit. B_{12}: 0.15 mcg

Creamy Sun-Dried Tomato Pasta

Silken tofu makes a creamy low-fat sauce base. If using dried tomatoes rather than oil-packed, be sure to rehydrate them well first. For another elegant twist on this dish, prepare this recipe with 1¼ cups chopped roasted red peppers instead of sun-dried tomatoes, or try a combination of the two. **Serves 4**

1 (12-oz.) package pasta	½ t. salt
1 block silken tofu, drained	1¼ c. sun-dried tomatoes, rehydrated
¼ c. soy milk	
2 T. red wine vinegar	1 t. parsley
½ t. garlic powder	2 T. chopped fresh basil

1. Cook pasta according to package instructions and drain well.
2. Blend together the tofu, soy milk, vinegar, garlic powder, and salt in a blender or food processor until smooth and creamy. Add tomatoes and parsley and pulse until tomatoes are finely diced.
3. Transfer sauce to a small pot and heat over medium-low heat just until hot.
4. Pour sauce over pasta and sprinkle with fresh chopped basil.

Animal Agriculture Affects Everyone
The powerful cocktail of hormones and antibiotics pumped into cows and chickens by today's food industry ends up right back in local water supplies and affects everyone, even vegans. All these antibiotics, combined with the cramped conditions of modern farms, lead to dangerous new drug-resistant pathogens and bacterial strains. Swine flu, bird flu, SARS, and mad cow disease are all traced back to intense animal agriculture practices.

Glasses of Water Consumed: _____

Thoughts About Today: _____

_____

_____

What I Ate Today

Time	Food Item	Amount	Calories	Fat	Carbs	Fiber	Protein
TOTAL							

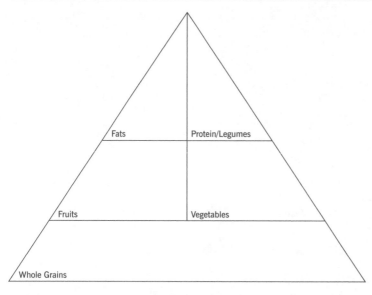

Friday

Breakfast

Breakfast wrap with 1 T. almond butter and ⅓ c. granola in a flour tortilla, 1 small apple, 1 c. orange juice

Cal.: 607.4; Fat: 15.7 g; Protein: 17.1 g; Sodium: 417.6 mg; Fiber: 10.9 g; Carbs.: 112.2 g; Sugar: 50.6 g; Zinc: 2.1 mg; Calcium: 448.1 mg; Iron: 3.98 mg; Vit. D: 2.7 mcg; Vit. B$_{12}$: 3 mcg

Lunch

½ c. baked beans with 1 veggie hot dog, 1 c. pineapple, 1 c. chocolate soy milk

Cal.: 402.5; Fat: 5.2 g; Protein: 22.9 g; Sodium: 1011.7 mg; Fiber: 14.3 g; Carbs.: 69.6 g; Sugar: 41.3 g; Zinc: 2.9 mg; Calcium: 363.5 mg; Iron: 8.28 mg; Vit. D: 0 mcg; Vit. B$_{12}$: 3 mcg

Snack

1 pita with 2 T. hummus

Cal.: 215; Fat: 3.5 g; Protein: 7.9 g; Sodium: 435.6 mg; Fiber: 3.1 g; Carbs.: 37.6 g; Sugar: 0.8 g; Zinc: 1.1 mg; Calcium: 63 mg; Iron: 2.4 mg; Vit. D: 0 mcg; Vit. B$_{12}$: 0 mcg

Dinner

10½ oz. No Shepherd, No Sheep Pie

Cal.: 345; Fat: 7.4 g; Protein: 18 g; Sodium: 553 mg; Fiber: 9.2 g; Carbs.: 53 g; Sugar: 2 g; Zinc: 5.7mg; Calcium: 129 mg; Iron: 5.4 mg; Vit. D: 0 mcg; Vit. B$_{12}$: 0.2 mcg

No Shepherd, No Sheep Pie

Sheep- and shepherd-less pie is a hearty vegetarian entrée for big appetites! **Serves 6**

1½ c. TVP	½ c. + 3 T. soy milk
1½ c. hot water or vegetable broth	1 T. flour
	5 medium potatoes, cooked
½ onion, chopped	2 T. vegan margarine
2 cloves garlic, minced	¼ t. rosemary
1 large carrot, sliced thin	¼ t. sage
2 t. oil	½ t. paprika (optional)
¾ c. sliced mushrooms	½ t. salt
½ c. green peas	¼ t. black pepper
½ c. vegetable broth	

1. Preheat oven to 350°F.
2. Combine TVP and hot water or vegetable broth, and allow to sit for 6–7 minutes. Gently drain any excess moisture.
3. In a large skillet, sauté onion, garlic, and carrot in oil until onion is soft, about 5 minutes. Add mushrooms, green peas, vegetable broth, and ½ cup soy milk. Whisk in flour just until sauce thickens, then transfer to a casserole dish.
4. Mash together the potatoes, margarine, and 3 T. soy milk with the rosemary, sage, paprika, salt and pepper, and spread over the vegetables.

Friday

Glasses of Water Consumed: _____

Thoughts About Today: _____

_____

_____

What I Ate Today

Time	Food Item	Amount	Calories	Fat	Carbs	Fiber	Protein
TOTAL							

Did you know? As a vegan, you personally save the lives of approximately eighty-three animals a year, reduce your carbon output by an average of 3,000 pounds, and conserve 1.4 million gallons of water a year. Now that's something to be proud of.

Saturday

Breakfast

1½ c. Chili Masala Tofu Scramble (See recipe in Week 2, Sat.)

Cal.: 418; Fat: 28 g; Protein: 29 g; Sodium: 527 mg; Fiber: 5.4 g; Carbs.: 16 g; Sugar: 2 g; Zinc: 3.6 mg; Calcium: 1125 mg; Iron: 6.5 mg; Vit. D: 0 mcg; Vit. B$_{12}$: 0 mcg

Lunch

Quesadillas with 2 oz. vegan cheese, 2 oz. chicken substitute, and ¼ c. broccoli in a flour tortilla, ½ c. black beans

Cal.: 358.5; Fat: 6.57 g; Protein: 17.05 g; Sodium: 444.75mg; Fiber: 12.43 g; Carbs.: 61.72 g; Sugar: 1.9g; Zinc: 1.55 mg; Calcium: 379.52 mg; Iron: 4.95 mg; Vit. D: 0 mcg; Vit. B$_{12}$: 0 mcg

Snack

Mixed fruit salad with ½ apple, ½ banana, ½ c. strawberries and ½ c. pineapple, granola bar (about 150 calories), 1 oz. cashews

Record nutritional values for your choice of granola bar in today's journal. The nutritional values below are for the mixed fruit salad and cashews only.

Cal.: 304.25; Fat: 12.95 g; Protein: 6.8 g; Sodium: 6.25 mg; Fiber: 6.65 g; Carbs.: 47.7 g; Sugar: 27.7g; Zinc: 1.95mg; Calcium: 40.3 mg; Iron: 2.7 mg; Vit. D: 0 mcg; Vit. B$_{12}$: 0 mcg

Dinner

5 oz. Quick Seitan Teriyaki Chow Mein

Cal.: 286; Fat: 19 g; Protein: 8.1 g; Sodium: 472 mg; Fiber: 2.5 g; Carbs.: 25 g; Sugar: 1.4 g; Zinc: 0.63 mg; Calcium: 39 mg; Iron: 3.1 mg; Vit. D: 0 mcg; Vit. B$_{12}$: 0 mcg

Quick Seitan Teriyaki Chow Mein

Serves 2

½ c. seitan, chopped

2 T. olive oil

¼ c. onion, sliced

½ green bell pepper, sliced into strips

½ red bell pepper, sliced into strips

¾ c. mushrooms, sliced

½ c. bean sprouts

1 (4-oz.) package chow mein noodles, prepared according to package instructions

2 T. soy sauce

2 T. teriyaki sauce

½ t. dash sesame oil

1. Brown seitan in olive oil for 3–5 minutes, then add onion, peppers, and mushrooms and heat, stirring frequently, until soft, another 3–5 minutes.

2. Add bean sprouts and allow to cook for 1 minute, then add noodles, soy sauce, teriyaki sauce, and sesame oil, gently mixing to combine. Cook for another minute, just until noodles are heated through.

Why Do Vegans Love Tofu So Much? Aside from low cost and ease of preparation, tofu is beloved by vegans as an excellent source of protein, calcium, and iron. Plain sautéed tofu with a dash of salt is a quick addition to just about any meal, and many grocery stores offer pre-marinated and even pre-baked tofu that is ready-to-go out of the package. What's not to love?

Glasses of Water Consumed: _____

Thoughts About Today: _____

_____

_____

What I Ate Today

Time	Food Item	Amount	Calories	Fat	Carbs	Fiber	Protein
TOTAL							

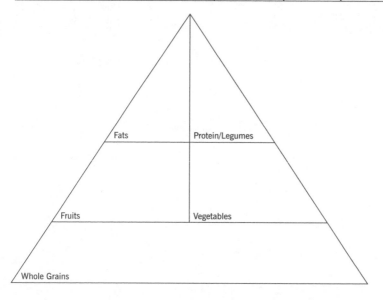

Sunday

Breakfast

Oatmeal breakfast bowl with 1 c. oatmeal, 1 c. blueberries, 1 oz. pecans, and 2 t. maple syrup

Cal.: 462.33; Fat: 24 g; Protein: 8.7 g; Sodium: 2.7 mg; Fiber: 10.3 g; Carbs.: 62.26 g; Sugar: 25.29 g; Zinc: 2.05 mg; Calcium: 37.43 mg; Iron: 2.06 mg; Vit. D: 0 mcg; Vit. B$_{12}$: 0 mcg

Snack

1 c. Crispy Baked Kale Chips (see recipe in Week 5, Sun.)

Cal.: 178; Fat: 9.3 g; Protein: 7.7 g; Sodium: 614 mg; Fiber: 4.4 g; Carbs.: 22 g; Sugar: 0 g; Zinc: 0 mg; Calcium: 292 mg; Iron: 4.5 mg; Vit. D: 0 mcg; Vit. B$_{12}$: 0.05 mcg

Lunch

Eggless Egg Salad sandwich (see recipe in Week 4, Mon.), with ¼ medium tomato, sliced, 2 slices whole grain bread, and ½ c. romaine lettuce

Cal.: 322.73; Fat: 14.3 g; Protein: 18.58 g; Sodium: 502.55 mg; Fiber: 6.38 g; Carbs.: 33.25 g; Sugar: 7.5 g; Zinc: 2.1 mg; Calcium: 452.03 mg; Iron: 3.73 mg; Vit. D: 0 mcg; Vit. B$_{12}$: 0 mcg

Dinner

Your choice! Choose a meal with about 450 calories (or less) and enjoy it with a slice of Chocolate Peanut Butter Explosion Pie

Record nutritional values for your dinner in today's journal. The nutritional values below are for the Chocolate Peanut Butter Explosion Pie only.

Cal.: 372; Fat: 23 g; Protein: 7.5 g; Sodium: 777 mg; Fiber: 1.4 g; Carbs.: 38 g; Sugar: 24 g; Zinc: 1 mg; Calcium: 32 mg; Iron: 1.4 mg; Vit. D: 0 mcg; Vit. B$_{12}$: 0.45 mcg

Chocolate Peanut Butter Explosion Pie

You can pretend it's healthy because it's made with tofu, or toss away all your troubles to the wind and just enjoy it. You'll feel like a kid again. **Serves 8**

¾ c. vegan chocolate chips

1 (12-oz.) block silken tofu

½ c. peanut butter

2 T. soy milk

1 prepared vegan cookie piecrust

1. Over very low heat or in a double broiler, melt the chocolate chips.
2. In a blender, puree tofu, peanut butter, and soy milk until combined, then add melted chocolate chips until smooth and creamy.
3. Pour into piecrust and chill for 1 hour, or until firm.

Glasses of Water Consumed: _____

Thoughts About Today: _____

_____

_____

What I Ate Today

Time	Food Item	Amount	Calories	Fat	Carbs	Fiber	Protein
TOTAL							

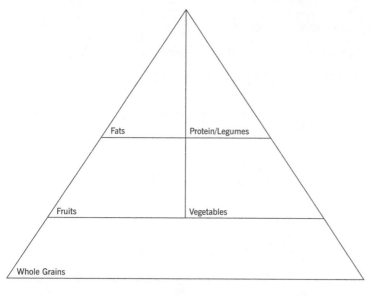

Fats

Protein/Legumes

Fruits

Vegetables

Whole Grains

WEEK 12 IN REVIEW

I feel: _____

_____

_____

_____

_____

My greatest food discovery this week was: _____

_____

_____

_____

This week's biggest vegan challenge was: _____

_____

_____

_____

New food I'd like to try: _____

_____

_____

_____

When I look back at this week, I most want to remember: _____

_____

_____

_____

Nutrition Totals

	Calories	Fat	Carbs	Fiber	Protein
Goal					
Actual					

Index